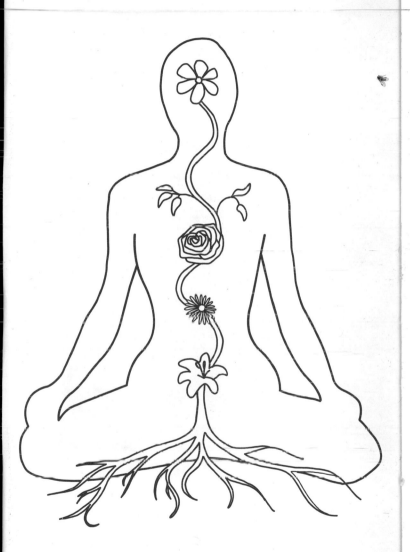

THE POWER
SOURCE

The POWER SOURCE

The Hidden Key to Ignite Your Core,
Empower Your Body,
Release Stress,
and Realign Your Life

LAUREN ROXBURGH

with a foreword
by Emmy Rossum

**goop
press**

GRAND CENTRAL
PUBLISHING

NEW YORK   BOSTON

Copyright © 2019 by Lauren Roxburgh

Cover design by Lisa Forde. Cover photography © 2018 Annie McElwain Ainsley. Cover copyright © 2018 by Hachette Book Group, Inc.

Grand Central Publishing
Hachette Book Group
1290 Avenue of the Americas, New York, NY 10104
grandcentralpublishing.com
twitter.com/grandcentralpub

First Edition: May 2019

Grand Central Publishing is a division of Hachette Book Group, Inc. The Grand Central Publishing name and logo is a trademark of Hachette Book Group, Inc.

The publisher is not responsible for websites (or their content) that are not owned by the publisher.

The Hachette Speakers Bureau provides a wide range of authors for speaking events. To find out more, go to www.hachettespeakersbureau.com or call (866) 376-6591.

Photography © 2018 Annie McElwain Ainsley

Art on page ii by Kelsey Vest

LCCN: 2019932505

ISBNs: 978-1-5387-6396-4 (hardcover), 978-1-5387-4892-3 (ebook)

Printed in the United States of America

LSC-C

10 9 8 7 6 5 4 3 2

*I dedicate this book with love to my adored husband,
Gus Roxburgh,
and our strong, vibrant daughters, Cameron and James.*

*. . . And to you, dear reader, may you awaken your pelvic
floor, personal power, and self love to prepare for
magic!*

Contents

Foreword

In the spring of last year, I was looking for a change. I had spent more than a decade pushing myself through grueling workouts, judging my body, comparing myself to others, and always feeling dissatisfied. More often than not, these intense sweat sessions left me feeling depleted, in pain, and down on myself. I was sure that only the most competitive, calorie-torching workouts could give me the results I desired. "No pain, no gain," I told myself. Massage, ice, and ibuprofen were the only counterpoints that could balance my body's response to the grueling routine I was in. The cycle was exhausting and I felt disconnected from my body.

It hadn't always been like this. I was a dancer as a teenager. Back then, I took such joy in movement. I loved my body. I loved what it could do, how strong I felt as I moved across the floor, how connected I felt to my core, how my muscles stretched and elongated. I began to realize that I was craving movement like that again—movement that made me feel better, not worse. How could I get back to that?

Enter Lauren Roxburgh. Initially I thought of her as The Roller Girl, and I must admit, I was skeptical. The idea of working out with a foam roller and squishy ball just didn't seem very challenging to me. I worried that giving up intense exercise would backfire on my waistline. But after an hour with Lauren, I was intrigued. At nearly six feet tall and with a big smile, Lauren radiates warmth, intelligence, and strength. She listens as much as she speaks. When we talked about movement, she used words like "fascia," "lymph system," and "pelvic floor," all of which were foreign concepts to me at the time. But for some reason, I immediately trusted her.

Through our work, I began to release layers of knotty tissue and restore blood flow to stagnant areas of my body. As my jaw loosened, my mind felt calmer. As I awakened my lymph system through graceful movement, rebounding, and self-care, I watched my skin texture smooth out. As I released the pressure on my diaphragm, I felt my anxiety lessen. As we broke up the knotty tissue in my shoulders, my arms lengthened and toned and my shoulders dropped. As my hip flexors started to open, the lean dancer legs I had loved as a teenager began to reveal themselves once again. As my pelvic floor released, I felt years of buried trauma unwind. I began to feel more connected to my own sensuality.

Lauren's movements are nurturing and replenishing. Instead of feeling drained after a punishing workout I didn't enjoy, I was suddenly looking forward to my rolling and rebounding sessions. It became a kind of therapy. I would bring my roller wherever I traveled, to hotels across the country and to my trailer on set. My joy in movement was restored. I felt good again.

Then came the affirmations. At first, I could only laugh. Lauren told me that anytime I had a negative thought about my body, I was to say aloud: "I live in the body of my dreams." At first, this felt ridiculous, comical, and uncomfortable. But I had trusted Lauren before and it had worked, so I agreed to try. Each time I'd experience negative self-talk and the anxiety that came with it, I'd shake it off and say aloud, "I live in the body of my dreams." This happened once in the supermarket and a woman buying broccoli nearby gave me a kind of quizzical smile and nod. Anyway, it works. See, your brain believes what you tell it. If you tell your brain, "you'll never be good enough," "you'll never be worthy," "you'll never have the body you want," or "you shouldn't feel empowered in your sensuality," well, that's what you'll believe. When you start to talk to yourself in a kind, supportive manner (and as if what you desire is already true), you reduce anxiety, reprogram your brain, release stress, and lower cortisol. With that, your body actually starts to change.

My friends began to say things like "you seem different" and "your energy is calmer, more centered." I was standing taller, unafraid to take up space in the room, while also feeling less reactionary and less judgmental of myself and others. I've gone down a jean size since I started working with Lauren, but that's not the best part. I feel stronger and more connected to my body than ever. I feel happy in my skin.

See, it's not about working hard—even though this work is hard—it's about working smart. It's about working *with* your body, not against it. The exercises in this book are gentle, but they reduce inflammation, work the fascia, and stretch the tissues in your body to engage metabolism and settle anxiety. It doesn't happen overnight, but this program is effective and sustainable.

Now, I can understand if as you're reading this, you might be thinking, "This sounds silly." But chances are, if you're reading this, you're looking for a change. Maybe, like me, you're in pain and looking for an easier road to a better solution. Maybe you're sick of grueling workouts, feeling disconnected to your sensuality, or stuck in the mindset of "no pain, no gain." Well, now I say, "No pain? That's a good thing."

It's time to reconnect to your true self, find your real body, shed whatever is holding you back physically or mentally, and create more space within yourself. You will be amazed when you see the beautiful body that exists underneath those layers of tension. I believe in the power of alignment and I'm so excited for you to experience the restorative, rejuvenating results that *The Power Source* can bring you.

—Emmy Rossum

Introduction

Before I could embrace my life and myself for who I really am—before I could let go of my notions of what "should be" and embrace what is—I was often disappointed and frustrated. I tried to control and hold on to everything. I had been an all-American swimmer and a collegiate athlete, so to many I was the epitome of "fitness." But my body was tight, heavy, and contracted, and so was my life. It wasn't until I learned to soften physically that I started to let go in other ways, too. I learned to change my perspective, harness stress, release stagnant emotions, and, most of all, let go of the need to control every situation. I learned how to surrender, let go of uphill battles, and stop trying too hard in general. With this, I began to live in a state of ease, gratitude, grace, acceptance, joy, and inner knowing.

I know all of this works, because I've created new patterns and habits in my body and my life. There was a time when my day-to-day life involved a lot of physical pain, tension, and fear. It felt like I was pushing to get through, both physically and emotionally. I didn't realize if I could just allow more, surrender, and go with the flow of life, everything in my life would improve—very much including my physical state.

Once I shifted my perspective, everything that I had been working so hard to change and struggling against fell into place easily. Equally importantly, the things that were not meant to be fell gently away without the anxiety or growing pains that I had been experiencing up to that point. I had found a better way to live in my own skin. With that, everything in my life transformed. *I* transformed.

We are all meant to receive the many gifts life has to offer. The problem is that, too often, we get in our own way by getting stuck in a story, belief system, or program. When we do this, we shut the door on possibility and get stuck in the way we think things are supposed to be. All we really accomplish when we do this is to create blockage, tension, more of the same story, more lack, and more exhaustion.

When people use phrases like "let go," "be vulnerable," or "get comfortable in your own skin," it can sound very nebulous. But there are actually things you can do in a pragmatic way and on an everyday basis that will get you there without a long to-do list. Not only that, but it's probably simpler than you think. The whole point here is to deepen your awareness, open up to possibilities, soften into your amazing self, become more present, and surrender to and embrace the flow of life instead of clutching to try to make things happen.

Surrender to Grace and Strength

If you have picked up this book, my guess is that you're looking for answers you have not yet found.

Perhaps you are experiencing ongoing or regular physical pain, inflammation, bloating, disconnection to your body, or tension. This might include lower back, neck, or jaw pain, or pain during sex. Maybe you are experiencing some sort of inflammation in the gut, the annoying feeling of perpetual bloat, a weak pelvic floor, or the inability to shed weight. You might be unable to take a deep breath. This might manifest emotionally as well, either as anxiety or depression or a feeling of perpetually ongoing stress or guilt. Or perhaps you're feeling something more nebulous than this—a nagging feeling that you have somehow veered off of the path that is meant for you. Only you're not sure what that path is or how to get back on it. Because of this, you might feel the need to grip and control rather than live in a state of gratitude, allowance, and grace.

Like so many of us, you may be living in a constant state of "white-knuckling" it and bearing down in your body and your life. This can manifest in both the very literal sense of creating tension and tightness in your body by clutching, and in the emotional sense of trying to hold on to or will a state of being rather than accepting and loving who and where you are.

Life has its up and downs, and when we try to live up to perfection (which does not exist), try to be someone we are not, or attempt to fit into someone else's box, it makes everything tenser, denser, and locked up. Quite frankly, it's exhausting. We become disconnected from ourselves, our purpose, from the world, and from our life. It affects us in very real ways on every level.

The goal here is to allow yourself to effortlessly and gracefully live in your amazing body and experience the life that you truly desire without *forcing* that life into being. But first, you have to define the life you want and align with your authentic self. It is only with this that everything else falls away. In order to understand what you want your life to be, you have to be able to make the space within yourself to listen and connect. You have to be able to feel and listen beyond the stress and pressure and hurdles of daily life and really understand what is going on inside. You have to be able to hear *you*. You have to choose to let go of the controlling and clutching and just *be* the beautiful person that exists underneath all of the negative self-talk and density.

This applies just as much physically as it does emotionally and energetically. Just as many of us live lives that are muted by stress, pressure, and stagnant emotion, many of our bodies have become physically altered by stress and clutching. For some of us, this manifests in the form of extra pounds that just won't come off, no matter what. For others, it manifests in the form of tension, knots, and pain. For some, it even presents itself in the form of disease. In this book, you will learn how to release the thick, dense armor of tension that often presents itself in our connective tissue. It is in our layer of connective tissue that we store up all of the unreleased physical and emotional energy that's built up over the years. With awareness and a few simple daily shifts, you will be able to experience freedom, fluidity, space, and lightness on a very physical level. It is difficult to imagine how freeing this is. But soon, you will see for yourself.

In the pages that follow, I will show you how to awaken your senses in order to bring yourself into the present moment. You will awaken to feeling, moving, smelling, and tasting. The tools in this book are designed to help revive your true essence, unlock your pure potential, and allow you to experience both the power of being present and the power of yourself. This is an inside job. Only you can do it. Once you do, you will build an awareness that will allow you to attract the right people, experiences, and relationships into your life. You will learn to lead with your heart to create tangible shifts in your body and in your life.

We live so much of our lives from a subconscious state. We have developed patterns, programs, brain loops, and habits that are on autopilot. It's like when you drive your car—you don't have to think about steering or braking; you just do it. The only way to make any changes in your body, in your surroundings, and in your life is by connecting to your deep subconscious. We connect to this part of our being through presence and inner silence. Our brains produce electrical patterns called brain waves, and new research has found that when we get into a slower, calmer, quieter state, we have more access to the subconscious mind and can make the positive adjustments we need to up-level in all areas of our life.

Think about it like this: your conscious mind governs your thoughts, and your subconscious mind governs your feelings. In order to create real, long-lasting, transformational change, your body, thoughts, emotions, and actions have to match your intentions. Your conscious and subconscious have to work together. You have to not just think about your intentions, but also *feel* them on a cellular level. Only then can a shift occur.

If you decide, for instance, that you are going to develop the habit of practicing 10 minutes of meditation every morning, and you truly commit to make the choice to invest in yourself, you can build that habit by meditating each morning until it becomes a subconscious program like brushing your teeth every morning. But if you just think, "Maybe I should meditate," and leave it at that, chances are that it won't become a part of your daily ritual. You are attempting to work solely from your conscious mind, without integrating the practice on a subconscious level.

In this book, you will build a new foundation from the inside out to merge together your conscious and subconscious. This includes a combination of mental and physical practices, mindfulness, and even some alternative therapy. The information you'll learn about is drawn from both Western and Eastern thought, bridging science with spirituality. You will learn to focus your perspective in the most positive direction, live more authentically, breathe more deeply, harness stress into motivation, and strengthen your pelvic floor (this might sound oddly specific, but very soon we'll discuss why this area of the body is critical to holistic wellness). You will become conscious of those things you can change for a rejuvenated body and a more fluid life of ease, joy, and purpose. From there, we will begin to develop subconscious habits through a series of awareness practices and presence.

Why the Pelvic Floor?

My mother was a model and actress who was quite focused on her physical appearance. Growing up around this, it's no surprise that from the time I was a teenager on, I was very body-focused. As an athlete, I was on a constant quest to build strength and embody physical fitness. The type of strength I built was forceful and dense. It didn't feel right for me, even though I made a conscious decision to build this strength, and went to a lot of effort to do so.

In my late twenties, I began studying structural integration, a form of alternative medicine that focuses on the body's connective tissue (also known as fascia). This was a game-changer for me. When I was doing my training, a teacher told me I had one of the tightest jaws and pelvic floors he had ever seen. Knowing what I know now, this isn't surprising. Aside from all of the force-ful workouts I was doing, I was also in an unhealthy marriage, my mother was deathly ill with cancer, and my business was experiencing major financial issues.

Most of the time, I didn't feel very good; I was incessantly stiff and tight. Everything in my body had locked up because of the combination of the hardcore workouts I was doing and the tension in my life. It was during structural integration training that I realized I was making choices for the outer world and not living authentically from my heart and gut. I started deepening my practices of self-care and learning more about how we as humans are all connected and how everything is energy. I started studying quantum physics and the law of attraction. It was then that the lightbulb went off. I realized that thoughts become things, energy attracts like energy, and we are so much more powerful than we are led to believe.

A few days after my mother passed away in 2010 (right around the same time I received my credentials as a structural integration practitioner), I felt led by my mom's spirit to an amazing bookstore in Topanga called Inn at the Seventh Ray. The book *Anatomy of the Spirit* by Caroline Myss literally fell off the shelf in front of me. It completely changed my life and my perspective on how powerful our emotions are, especially when it comes to the health and vitality of our bodies and our true fulfillment in life. My focus shifted to the body-mind-heart connection and holistic healing. Whereas the work I had been doing with clients previously centered completely on their physical health, I now began to help them work on their emotional wealth, as well. I focused on healing and looking within to view the body and wellness from a holistic perspective.

As I dove deeper into the physical, mental, and emotional mechanics and connections within the human body, it became more and more clear to me how incredibly important the pelvic floor is. I also began noticing the state of my clients' pelvic floor and how it related to other issues in their bodies and emotional lives. Because so many of us have lost our connection to this powerful area of our body, we've also lost the ability to mindfully relax the area. Without connection, we also lose sensation, tone, resilience, and flexibility in the pelvic floor. When we can't connect to our pelvic floor, we also cannot connect to our deep core muscles. This certainly makes it more difficult to feel and tone our bodies, but it also makes us weaker and sets off a whole chain of reactions—biological, neurological, and emotional—that inhibit us from attaining vibrant holistic wellness.

When we lose the connection to those deep muscles, it becomes difficult to relax the area. This means that the pelvic floor becomes hypertonic, or perma-flexed. Imagine flexing your bicep constantly and never fully letting go: the muscles will become weak, exhausted, and disconnected. That's what most of us are doing with our pelvic floor all of the time. If you did this same thing to your bicep muscle, after a while, you would lose flexibility, strength, and the ability to relax. That's more or less what happens to the pelvic floor. Until, that is, you become aware of the stress and tension in the area and do some work to alleviate it. Part of this is willfully relaxing and unclenching these muscles—and then directing energy to build strength.

In Eastern traditions, the pelvic floor is known as the root chakra—it's where we hold our fears; specifically fears around primary instincts, such as our health, our family's safety, and our financial security. It's where we process emotion and house our fight-or-flight reactions. You know that feeling when you get cut off by someone while driving, get bad news, or are about to go into a high-stress situation? This can cause you to clench your pelvic floor.

We talk about holistic health all of the time, but we never talk about the pelvic floor. If we don't bring the pelvic floor into the discussion, it's not really holistic health at all. We are missing out on an entire, very critical area and energy of the body, one that has a serious impact on our physical, emotional, and energetic wellness.

In 2014, I published an article in *goop* about what I had come to realize in terms of the relationship between the pelvic floor, mind-body connection, fascia, and stress. I was stunned by the response and by how many people—particularly women—related to what I was talking about.

The floodgates opened. People flew in to work with me from all over the world, and the volume of clients was so intense I had to refer them out to other practitioners. At the time, there were very few bodyworkers or physical therapists who understood the mind-body connection as it pertains to the pelvic floor. Four years later, that is beginning to change.

It's not that *no one* has ever addressed holistic health through the lens of the pelvic floor. They have, just not to the masses in America. In France, for example, health insurance has long covered pelvic floor rehabilitation following childbirth. We are behind other areas of the world in this regard, and it's time we catch up. Too many women struggle with incontinence, pelvic pain, inability to have an orgasm, low back pain, a weak deep core, the dreaded post-baby pooch, middle-aged pooch, and pain during sex. And these are only the examples of issues that are *clearly* related to the pelvic floor. There is so much more. The health of our pelvic floor has a significant trickle-down effect on the health of our entire body, being, and emotional life.

Today, my practice focuses on personal development, empowerment, and alignment of all areas of life and being. My intention is to help us all shift the paradigm that says we need to abuse our bodies and ourselves in order to see results. In both my own life and through working with clients, I have come to believe that we only truly see results through emotionally choosing to transform and actually nourishing and nurturing ourselves. Of course, this sounds obvious, but it is not a practice that most Americans engage in.

The end result of this work is that clients have a huge shift. They come to a place of inner knowing, feeling more, allowing the good to flood in, acceptance, grace, and flow. They experience an empowering change in mindset that allows them to get out of the adrenal fatigue stress mode and into a thriving, present, connected state. They begin to reset, feel incredible in their bodies, and live with more purpose and gratitude.

As human beings, we are not meant to be in a state of doing all of the time. Nourishing, nurturing, allowing, listening, and cleansing will always get you to your end result more happily and effectively than clutching, fighting, controlling, and forcing. We want to get into the flow, rather than fighting against resistance.

A Quick Shout-Out to You Mamas: Pelvic Floor Recovery for Pregnancy and Labor

For many women, the experience of childbirth might be the first time you ever hear the term "pelvic floor." And since the pelvic

floor is at the heart of everything we will discuss in the coming pages, it's important to address how this area of the body is
impacted during the journey of pregnancy and labor—because
there's no doubt that having a baby can do a number on your
entire system and, of course, the pelvic floor. (Please note that
all of the tools and information in this book will still apply to
you, regardless of gender and whether or not you have ever given
birth.)

The muscles, tissues, and nerves of your pelvic floor are
stretched and pressed down during pregnancy due to the weight
of your baby. This is compounded by a flood of the hormone
relaxin, which allows you to stretch even more. This is only
the beginning. During childbirth, your pelvic floor opens and
expands, which after pregnancy and birthing can result in scar
tissue (which is considerably denser than regular tissue), trauma,
and damage to the nerve endings in this region. In short, your
body—particularly your pelvic floor—goes through a lot to
miraculously give birth.

In France, insurance pays for postnatal pelvic floor therapy.
Here in America, we don't offer much to postnatal women after
their 6-week postpartum OB-GYN visit. Even at this, doctors are
primarily monitoring your ovaries, not your pelvic floor. No one
tells us how to heal the pelvic floor or, for that matter, that we
even need to heal, restore, and reconnect to our pelvic floor. No
one talks about how a pelvic floor that is not restored will go on
to impact the rest of the body in all the ways we are discussing
throughout this book.

Every woman requires a recovery period after giving birth,
which should last for a minimum of 6 to 8 weeks postdelivery.
During this period, most women experience sensations ranging

from discomfort to pain, along with incontinence, which is normal. For all of us, this should be a period of healing and rest that involves physical exertion no greater than a bit of light walking.

If after these first several weeks you experience ongoing incontinence, lower back pain, or tightness in your hips, it's a sign your pelvic floor has not healed or has healed incorrectly. Unfortunately, many women think this is their new status quo. It doesn't have to be!

I've had many clients tell me they were informed that incontinence is just something they have to deal and live with postbirth. This is absolutely not the case. In fact, I've helped these same clients heal through a combination of body awareness, pelvic core connection, contract and relax Kegels, deep squats, body rolling, gentle bouncing, and diaphragmatic breathing.

The good news is that, although they're not widely discussed, there are actually more opportunities now than ever before for postnatal pelvic floor recovery. Among these are postnatal yoga, light bouncing on the rebounder, Pilates classes and physical therapists who specialize in the pelvic floor, and even online programs that focus on pelvic floor recovery.

The reality is that everyone's pelvic floor health should be checked and monitored post-childbirth. We're not there yet—but with these modalities, we're moving in the right direction.

I don't teach anything I don't practice. For me, it was motherhood that brought about the type of transformation I'll share with you in this book. Being with my daughters drew me further into the present moment. I was making a concerted effort to really be with my children, and in doing so, I simultaneously was with and learned a lot about myself as well. I wanted to parent from a calm, loving, conscious place, and so I first chose to figure out a way to get myself to that place. Before my daughters came along, I had lived my life on a hamster wheel. I never had time; I was always busy, stressed, and in a rush. I constantly experienced tension and pain, and generally felt thicker, denser, heavier, and exhausted.

Of course, you don't have to be a parent to have this transformative experience. All you have to do is make a decision. You have to decide to get out of survival mode and into a place of healing, thriving, and creating. Getting to this place is based purely on choice. Today, most of us default to stress and busyness or even become a victim to them. We live in a society where stress has become an excuse to avoid dealing with things like our true, authentic feelings. The truth is, we always have choice. Stress is a choice, although if we make that choice enough over time it becomes a subconscious reaction, and we lead our lives in a state of fear. There is a direct correlation between stress and fear because stress is a fight-or-flight response. We were designed to feel stress as a way for our cavemen ancestors to survive. When our body feels stress, it interprets it as fear.

You get to choose how you react to any given situation. You get to choose what you do with your life on a daily basis. It might not always feel like it, but the truth is that the power is always in your hands. But before you can connect with that, you first have to make the choice to tune in, become aware and present, listen to your inner feelings, and reconnect with yourself. This is a choice that you will continue to make on a second-by-second basis until, after a while, it's no longer a choice. Instead, it's a way of living and feeling free.

Together, we are going to shift from survival mode into a place of ease, confidence, flow, and alignment. But first, you have to make that choice. I'm also going to give you some simple and practical tools to heal your pelvic floor if you have had a baby—and the good news is this is a remarkably resilient part of the body with almost miraculous powers of recovery.

What to Expect

The truth is, there are many different and equally valid ways to look at life and the world. I find that the more open I can be to various philosophies and schools of thought, the richer my life experience becomes. In my practice, I straddle both Western and Eastern thought, and my passion is to integrate science with spirituality. I am fascinated by the biology of the body, but I also believe we are energetic beings and that holistic and integrative medicinal practices can heal us. When we extract different elements from various schools of thought, we can begin to heal, strengthen, and align our bodies and entire systems in a holistic way, inside and out.

You don't have to change the circumstances of your life to enhance how you feel and how you experience life. It's about reframing how you *feel* about where you are and what you have *right now* and believing in infinite possibilities. That is a quantum shift that will allow good to flow in. More good than you can probably even imagine right now.

Together, we will work our way through each area of the body, beginning with the pelvic floor. We will discuss how the pelvic floor impacts each of the other areas and how we uniquely hold tension, fear, and stress in each area. I will explain how this impacts us physically, emotionally, and energetically. Most exciting of all, I will also explain the distinct superpowers that are held within each area of the body and show you the keys for unlocking them. I will help you remove the blockages, fears, tensions, and inflammation that are weighing you down, and replace them with power, strength, confidence, robust energy, and motivation.

This book will bring you into the present moment by awakening your senses. The tools included within these pages will help you start feeling your bodily sensations again, which will help you make more empowered choices and release heavy emotional baggage and unnecessary tension. You will begin to understand you have very real superpowers you never even realized were there. You will learn that the only things you can control are your reactions and choices, and you will begin to make more empowered choices that add a greater sense of ease to your daily life and improve both your physical and emotional life.

1

It All Begins with the Pelvic Floor

Not too long ago, I fell into a conversation with a woman I had just met at a dinner party. As is often the case when people find out what I do for a living, the discussion turned to some discomfort she was experiencing. This woman told me about a chronic knot in her shoulder that she could not get rid of. If you've ever experienced a knot of scar tissue in your shoulder (or anywhere else for that matter), you know exactly how annoying and frustrating they are. Can you live with it? Well, sure. But the discomfort is always there in the background, like an annoying hum that never goes away.

This woman had tried everything. She had been to a number of top-of-the line masseuses, body healers, physical therapists, and spas. She was consistent and relentless in her effort to get rid of this knot once and for all. No matter what modality she tried or practitioner she went to, nothing changed. That knot wasn't going anywhere.

"Let me try something," I told her.

I asked her to sit down and then moved behind her chair and rested my hands on her shoulders. "Now, do a Kegel by contracting your pelvic floor. Hold it and then slowly release, relax, and feel it open and soften. And now soften and relax one more layer," I said.

She paused for a brief moment at my request, as most people do. However, she was so desperate to get rid of the discomfort that had been plaguing her for so long I'm pretty sure this woman would have done anything I asked her to, no matter how "out there" it seemed.

She did the contraction and contrasting relaxation. I know this because I immediately felt her shoulders melt.

Like most people I work with, she was completely shocked. As far as she was concerned, I had spread some fairy dust over her or pulled some sort of knot-releasing magic out of a hat. She couldn't believe that after everything she had tried and all of the money she spent in the process, it was the simple awareness of the base of her core (the pelvic floor) and the neuromuscular connection a Kegel provides that ultimately alleviated her rigidity, pain, and discomfort.

What I'm doing isn't actually magic at all. Even better than that, it all boils down to science, biology, fascia, and the nervous system.

The Pelvic Floor Connection

The shoulders and jaw aren't the only parts of our body that are influenced by our connection to the pelvic floor. Our entire body is. More than that, our pelvic floor impacts not just our physical well-being, but also our emotional health. In fact, the pelvic floor lies at the very heart of this mind-body connection we hear so much about these days.

We'll get to *why* this is the case shortly. First, let's talk about the benefits as you begin the work of connecting, awakening, and healing your pelvic floor to align your body and your life. You will notice:

- increased flexibility
- a metabolism boost
- decreased lower back tension and pain
- a more relaxed face, brow, and jaw
- a deeper enjoyment of intimacy
- a flatter tummy
- a release of general tightness, including knots and persistent pain
- better range of motion
- improved digestion and immunity
- a longer, leaner physique
- rejuvenated, glowing skin

You can see why the tools in this book seem more like magic than science sometimes. While science and biology lie at the root of what we're about to discuss, what's most important here is awareness and *practice*. Before you can release and enhance the well-being of your pelvic floor, first you have to feel it and connect with it. Most of us are completely disconnected from this area of our body. As a result, we subconsciously clutch and hold a lot of tension and tightness there that effectively clog up our entire body in a chain reaction that works its way up to our cranium.

Alleviating this is simple enough once you know what to do, but it involves much more than just Kegels.

By the time you finish reading the pages that follow, you will understand how to connect with your pelvic floor—the first step in connecting with all of the other areas of your body. Reconnecting you with your body will connect you to presence and your true emotions, allowing you to process, harness, or release stress and awaken your core. With this, your holistic health will improve by leaps and bounds *and*—as if all of that isn't enough—you will even unlock a variety of superpowers you've been sitting on that I bet you didn't even know you had!

Incredible, right? So, let's get started, beginning with taking a look at why this works.

The Pelvic Floor and Holistic Health

Located at the base of our spine, the pelvic floor serves as our foundation. You can think of it much like the roots of a tree. In the chakra system, the first chakra, which governs the pelvic floor, is known as the root chakra. Just like a tree isn't as healthy, grounded, strong, stable, and nourished as it could be when its roots aren't strong, neither is the human body.

Most of us know that our core makes us strong. However, when we think of the core, we generally think of our abs and obliques. Our core actually starts down in the base of our pelvic floor, which is why I refer to the pelvic floor as the "pelvic core" in my practice. To have a strong, stable core, we have to begin with our incredible base, the pelvic floor. There's no way around it. No matter how many sit-ups or crunches you do, you're never going to build the strength, length, or the grace you desire without first awakening and creating resilience and flexible strength in your pelvic floor.

It is the pelvic floor that supports the core and organs. Just like a building can't stand on a weak foundation, such is the relationship between our pelvic floor and core. This analogy continues all the way up through the body, as each area (or power center, as I call them) stacks on top of the one before.

It's important to understand that the type of strength I'm talking about here isn't the sort of rigid, rock-hard, congested strength you build up at the gym. I'm talking about the sort of graceful and supple strength that promotes holistic, vibrant health. Rather than building up congestion in the muscles, we are going to elongate them and make them more flexible and resilient. This is a very specific type of strength, and one that we don't usually focus on cultivating. It will make your entire system more efficient and nimble. *This* is how our bodies were meant to exist in their optimal state. We'll talk more about this shortly.

The Pelvic Floor and Life Force

Many of us today are completely unaware of and disconnected from these bodies we live our life in. We spend so much time in our head that we aren't fully grounded in our physicality. Because of this, we miss out on the nuances of what's happening within us and the messages from our body asking for change. Often, we don't even recognize when an area of our body is out of balance or needs a little extra TLC.

This is exacerbated by the fact that because we are holistic creatures, issues that originate in one area of the body may very well present or manifest themselves in other areas of the body. This can make the root cause of an issue very difficult to identify. Instead, we just know that we don't feel right—this might evidence itself in any number of ways, including lingering pain, chronic disease, weight gain, lethargy, anxiety, and a closed mind, among others.

In the Kundalini tradition—as well as many other Eastern philosophies—it is believed that the flow of life force energy, known as *chi*, begins in the pelvic region. Of course, this makes sense because creation of *life* begins in the pelvic area through the process of reproduction. Life force energy governs charisma, connection, and creation—all of the things that enliven us and make us human. From our pelvis, this energy flows up and animates all of the other power centers of our body—our deep core, upper core, heart, and head. This energy is meant to flow freely, system-wide.

Like any other type of energy, life force energy can become stuck or stagnant. This happens when we experience congestion or blockages, both physical and emotional. In the event an energy disruption occurs in one power center of our body, that life force is cut off and cannot flow freely to the other power centers. These blockages can occur anywhere between its origination point in the pelvis all the way up to our head. To experience maximum health, we must ensure that each area of our body is healthy, open, and free-flowing. Otherwise, it will create a break in the chain, so to speak.

The whole purpose of acupuncture is to unblock chi. Blocked chi can result in pain, disruption, and stagnation, both physical and emotional. When life force is freely flowing, all of our systems run more efficiently and effectively. We feel lighter and possess a greater sense of vitality. When our chi is flowing, we gravitate toward other freely-flowing life forces—for example, we nourish ourselves with better foods. (Plants and animals and all other organic beings contain life force as well, as does Earth itself.)

Together, we will engage in practices that enhance our sense of awareness and connection. With this, we will become more adept at preventing and identifying issues of clutching, tightness, and congestion so that we can create a free-flowing stream of beautiful and abundant life energy all the way from our pelvic floor up to the crown of our head.

Harnessing the Power Centers

Throughout our body, we have five primary power centers:

- pelvic floor
- deep core
- upper core
- heart and shoulders
- head, neck, and jaw

Each of these areas serves a distinct physical and biological function and relates to the endocrine system. Each area plays a role in helping regulate our hormones, metabolism, and brain function. In addition, each of them is also associated with specific emotions and elements of life.

It turns out that each of these power centers is also the seat of a unique superpower. These superpowers include: awakening our personal power, sensuality, confidence, love, and connection. No matter how you feel in this exact moment, the truth of the matter is that you are a powerful, exquisite creature. If you find one of these superpower qualities doesn't resonate with you at all, chances are that's a key indicator that it's in an area of the body that needs some attention, balance, and nourishing.

Throughout this book, we'll examine each of these superpowers, and you'll learn how to unlock them for maximum expression and results. You will be amazed at how your life begins to transform on every level once you bring them to full bloom. By aligning your body and your power centers, you will also align your choices, time, and, ultimately, your life. You will unearth and bring into the world the truest version of yourself by aligning your intentions with your actions—and you will feel empowered with the ability to identify, own, and walk the path that is uniquely yours.

The Pelvic Floor and Stress

Have you been around a baby recently? If so, maybe you've noticed how incredibly flexible and nimble they are. If you're a yogi, perhaps you've observed that babies naturally go into poses like the aptly named Happy Baby, Child's Pose, and even a shorter-armed version of Downward Dog.

There is a reason babies do this: their bodies are in their natural fluid state, which is flexible, strong, and resilient. This is how we were all designed to be. Not only do babies exist in a natural physical state, but they also exist in a natural emotional state—open, joyful, curious, and happy. On all levels, babies are unblocked and free-flowing. You started out that way, too. More than that, you have the ability to get back to this state. It's where your body, mind, and heart *truly* desire to be.

Over time, though, we build up congestion due to injuries; trauma; unfelt, unprocessed, or swallowed emotions; and the stresses of day-to-day life. We build up stagnant and blocked energy; we begin to live in a state of fight-or-flight, which makes it more difficult for our bodies to rest and heal. This is a self-perpetuating cycle. Once we hold stress, we acquire even more stress, because we get stuck in a pattern of contraction: we live in a reactive state and are unable to process and release all the tension and pressure, both physical and emotional.

When you get out of this crazy cycle, your body will reboot, you'll sleep more deeply, your sugar craving will diminish, your healing systems will work better, and your body will become more efficient and less stagnant. You won't get sick as often, because your immune system will be more robust with the alleviation of stress.

From an aesthetic standpoint, your belly will become flatter: science has shown us that pooched bellies are often correlated with excess stress and abdominal fat, particularly in women. This happens because excess weight is essentially excess energy stored as fat; it is the result of the adrenal fatigue that comes from stress. In addition, your skin will clear up, and your face will glow. This process will help your body become less inflamed or bloated and more flexible, which prevents premature aging. It will even tame your hunger hormones.

What does all of this have to do with the pelvic floor? Everything.

In the world today, we spend a lot of time talking about stress.

We talk about how stressed and busy we are. We talk about how we need to de-stress. Often, we even talk about specific ways to work toward a more stress-free existence. Still, most of us never break the cycle. We remain stuck here in a story, on the hamster wheel, growing more stressed out as each day goes by.

The reason we are stuck, and why none of these stress antidotes work, is because we are rarely treating the problem in a holistic way. We may try to target one area or treat one symptom, but the only way to achieve lasting change is by addressing the whole picture. Unfortunately, the pelvic floor's connection to the nervous system is rarely involved in the discussion. If we really want to avoid falling victim to stress in our lives—or, better yet, harness the energy used in the reaction we know as stress and channel it into motivation and empowerment—then the pelvic floor *has* to be at the very center of that conversation.

The Stress On/Off Button

Our nervous system is composed of a network that runs up and down our spinal cord, from our cranium to our sacrum. This is known as the craniosacral connection.

Powerful forces of fluid and energy run along our spinal nervous system, all the way from our sacrum, up our spinal cord to our brain, and back again. Our sacrum—the triangular bone at the base of the spine—is located directly above our pelvic floor. This means that if we want to manage stress, we have to combat it at the beginning of the network—you guessed it: the pelvic floor. You can think of this area of the body as housing our stress on/off button.

This button is flipped on and asks for a surge of energy when we react and clutch in our pelvic floor. Stress and clutching go hand-in-hand. When we are in a reactive state of stress, our natural biological reaction is to subconsciously clutch the pelvic floor. This clutching then sends out a system-wide message that throws our body into the sympathetic nervous system state of fight, fright, or flight, which accelerates the aging process, is exhausting, and makes us live in a reactive state.

Our cavemen ancestors needed this stress button for their literal life-or-death survival. When true danger loomed, they needed a hit of adrenaline to flee to safety. But the world is different now. We still have the stress button, and sometimes we *do* need it during those moments when we are in danger. However, most of us don't live our lives under constant life-or-death threat. The problem is that our bodies *think* we do because of this vicious unconscious clutching cycle. We live in a constant state of clutch and compression, so our bodies think we are under duress, and our fight-or-flight system kicks into gear. Constantly.

The busy-ness of the world exacerbates this problem even more. We clutch because we're stuck in traffic, because our inbox is jammed, because we're worried about money, or because we have too much to do and not enough time to do it. In response, we clutch, push through, try to make things happen, and attempt to control everything. Most of us are stuck here, and we don't even realize it. This pared-down, white-knuckling way of life has become the new normal.

Not only does this way of being feel terrible and exhausting, it also makes you feel like a victim of your own life. The good news is that it's much easier than you think to shift your perspective and channel the energy we've been dedicating toward stress in an entirely different, more joyful, and more beneficial direction.

When we are in an optimal, unstressed state, our parasympathetic system runs the show. It is from this state—and only from this state—that our bodies kick into rest-and-digest mode, which I believe is the fountain of youth. When we are in rest-and-digest, our bodies can flow into their true graceful and abundant potential, and we can connect to our inner voice, heal, and learn how to shift our perspective and adapt our reactions to the ups and downs that do occur in the course of life more fluidly.

Evolving

We live in a world of incredible technology and innovation. Every year, new inventions come into the world that change the fabric of our lives. Even at that, nothing we create will ever be as elegant, refined, or resilient as the human body. It is time that we make use of this incredible gift we've been given by empowering ourselves with knowledge and awareness about our miraculous bodies. By doing this, we can learn how to evolve our systems as our world evolves. We can make more empowered choices so that we do not fall victim to what we think of as the stresses of life. Instead, we can harness this energy, shift our mindset, advance our bodies and reactions, and learn how to thrive rather than just survive. The more you understand how your body works, the more prepared you will be to make better choices that will enhance the quality of your life and the vitality of your body.

The body is an amazing, orchestrated masterpiece that *wants* to be in its optimal state. It wants to be joyful, relaxed, passionate, and unstuck. The body is also an incredible communicator if you're willing to listen. When we feel pain or tension, it's usually the body alerting you to an issue, asking you to make a change, to let go of something, or to build strength somewhere. This book will give you the tools to do this.

All we have to do is tune in, feel more, be more responsible with our reactions and choices, and rewire the signals in our mind to shift our reality. Once we decide to live in a more empowered place by being more mindful of our time, choices, decisions, relationships, and accountability, everything begins to shift in the most incredible ways.

In the following pages, I am going to teach you how to work your way up from your center of creation by encouraging you to become more present and awaken your senses of feeling, hearing, smelling, seeing, and tasting. I will explain why this works and empower you with simple shifts that will have the greatest impact in the least amount of time. With this, you will cultivate awareness of and take control of your stress responses, and so much more.

You will also immerse yourself in the fountain of youth by decreasing the toxic hormones released from a constant reactive and "stressful" life. These reactive hormones can age us prematurely, lower our immune system, cause heart disease, damage our DNA and brain cells, and put us into a negative emotional state.

My intention in writing this book is to help you connect to a newfound strength, inner knowing, and confidence to create resilience in your physical body, and to guide you to a more enjoyable and elevated emotional state. You will be amazed as your body relaxes into a more aligned, vibrant version of itself. You will release old emotional baggage, your tension will begin to melt away, and you will feel more present, grateful, and elevated on all levels.

2

How It All Works

In life, it's easy to get stuck in certain ways of thinking and feeling. We label ourselves as a "type" of person and make our decisions from that place. It's wonderful to understand who we are; however, when we get too locked in to a limited and specific school of thought, we can miss out on new information and other ways of thinking, being, and living that might benefit and expand us and our experience in our bodies and lives.

As we discuss each power center of the body, we will look at it through both Western and Eastern lenses. Consider new ways of thinking about your body and mind-body connection. Take away what resonates with you, and don't worry about the material that doesn't.

Give Yourself Some Love

At the beginning of each chapter, you will find a summary of common physical and emotional symptoms that are present when that power center needs some connection, attention, and healing.

If you find yourself experiencing two or more of these symptoms, it likely means that you are experiencing some degree of blockage in that power center, and you will find the information and tools in that chapter to be of particular relevance to you.

You may very well find that you are experiencing some degree of imbalance in many or even all of the power centers. This is common, and not a cause for distress or shame. Remember that these power centers are intricately connected and build on top of one another. They are designed to help you connect to a deeper wealth of power that lies within you. If your pelvic floor is out of balance—and most of ours are—that will have an impact on all of the power centers that live above it as well.

Even if you find you are not experiencing any of the issues cited at the beginning of the chapter, many of these tools will still be useful to you in terms of bolstering your holistic health and becoming more attuned with and knowledgeable about your body. These power center run-downs will provide you with an easy way to identify where an imbalance or issue lives and to target it quickly and directly at the source. On your first read, I recommend that you look through the whole book and put into practice whatever resonates with you from each of the power centers. Once you start to experience the benefits, it will be even easier to start digging deeper into this practice—and hopefully your curiosity will be piqued enough that you'll want to try some of the therapies that are totally new to you!

The Imbalanced Power Center

Each chapter will include a case study from my own practice, demonstrating what issues within that power center look like in practice. I find it's always helpful to see how information impacts us in real-life ways, and that is precisely the intent of this section. It will also provide an overview of how a seemingly run-of-the-mill symptom is indicative of and at the root of other disparate issues in our life.

My favorite part of my work—and what I hope these case studies drive home—is the degree to which the information I'm sharing transforms life on every level. Sure, your aching jaw might be an annoyance on a day-to-day basis, but when you see how addressing that issue spirals out to have a profound impact on your ability to communicate and connect with the world and get in touch with your intuition, you will be floored.

Get to Know Your Physical Body

Our bodies are beautifully automated, so we often don't stop to think about how they work. Not only is it important to have a visual of what we're made of, but this understanding of the physicality of our body builds awareness and also helps us appreciate our bodies for the miraculous entities they are.

Holistic Health

This section of each chapter will explain how the power center interacts with and impacts other areas of the body. Here we also begin to understand how real and impactful our emotions actually are. For example, when someone experiences heartbreak, it generally leads to emotions like resentment and self-protection, emotions that are associated with the heart area. These emotions often manifest physically in the form of hunched shoulders. That, in turn, impacts the alignment of our entire upper body and impedes our breath. At a time when we most need to be in a healing mode, we become less able to work through our experience. This type of reaction can happen in many areas of the body.

Enhancing our connection with our body connects us to our emotions, allowing us to feel them, learn from them, and move through and process them in a healthy way. Certain emotions tend to "live" in certain areas of the body. When we become aware of what is happening physically, it often gives us clues about what is happening emotionally as well. The opposite can also be true.

When we follow the clues and messages our body provides about our emotional state, we can then begin to release stagnant emotions. This unblocks our energy and empowers us with access to a new resource of vigor and vibrancy. We live in a world that is largely focused on *doing*. However, we also want to create more time to just *be* in and enjoy our lives.

Our emotions exist for a reason. We are meant to feel them so we can act and live from an authentic place. When we don't feel our emotions, we can't work through and release them, so they fester and become stagnant and swallowed. Not only is this emotionally unhealthy and stress-inducing, but it also creates physical blockages within the body. These blockages can actually lead to physical suffering—whether that means developing a literal disease, or pain, discomfort, exhaustion, or unnecessary extra weight—and lowered life force energy. This is why what I like to call emotional hygiene is so important!

When I first started my journey in structural integration, I was in an unhealthy marriage. After my initial structural alignment session (which forms the foundation for much of the content you'll find in this book), I felt like I had been not only through intense physical therapy, but also intense *emotional* therapy. I walked away feeling empowered, like I could take on the world. Not surprisingly, my life changed for the better in monumental ways as I became more emotionally aware and integrated tools to more effectively process emotions.

Of course, there are other ways to get in touch with our emotions as well, such as talk therapy. While this can be a great solution for some, for others it's *too* much time in their heads. For some people, talk therapy on its own keeps them stuck in a feeling of victimization. This is not to say that talk therapy doesn't serve a purpose—it absolutely does. However, it's also important to know there's a complementary way to enhance your results or find relief in a different modality of healing altogether. That other way is precisely what we'll be learning about. I like to call it movement medicine. With this aligned life philosophy, you will empower yourself, take responsibility for your life and your well-being, and awaken the brilliant vitality and life force within you.

I totally get that it often feels easier to avoid emotions when they are difficult. Some of those will probably come up as you work your way through the power centers. Remember that the point here is ultimately to release those emotions for holistic health; I will provide you with the tools to do that.

Chakra Connection

It wasn't until I was well along in formulating my power center theory that I realized the power centers and chakras largely
match up (although there are seven chakras and only five power
centers). In each chapter, I will explain the chakra associated with
the power center to draw a richer picture of what's at stake and to
demonstrate how the ideas we're discussing in this book correlate
with Eastern philosophy.

Eastern philosophy holds that we have seven chakras (or energy
centers) spread throughout and around the body. These energy centers correlate with certain areas of our life, as well as emotional and
spiritual experience. Each chakra governs a different area of the body
as well as a specific aspect of life. For example, the root chakra, found
in the pelvic area, governs our sense of roots, family, survival, safety,
and our foundation.

It's also interesting to note that there is a correlation between
the placement of our glands and the chakra system. In Chinese
medicine, the seven chakras are connected to the different glands
in our body. When those chakra areas are out of alignment or
shut down, the glands are impacted, which influences our mood,
physical wellness, and general life force.

Eastern philosophy looks at this phenomenon from an energetic standpoint, while Western medicine looks at it from a physical standpoint—but both schools of thought boil down to the
same outcomes.

We will take a look at the chakra (or chakras) associated with
each power center. Some people really find themselves in the idea
of chakras, while others simply don't resonate with them. No

matter where you stand, the chakra system still provides us with information that is relevant and important to our understanding of the power center. If you don't find yourself connecting with the concept of chakras, don't worry—there are many different ways into the exercises of this book!

The Root Connection

We are each a living, breathing tapestry. Like a tapestry, our bodies are connected by a series of interwoven threads. This is a beautiful thing, but it sometimes means that pain and discomfort often present themselves in one area of the body but originate from another.

In this section, we will learn how to look at our bodies in global terms and to make sense of the different threads that compose each of our unique tapestries. As you come along with me on this journey, I will explain how each power center is related to the pelvic floor, how the power centers work together, and how one impacts the other.

Stress

The stress reaction has the ability to live in every area of our body. In each place, it manifests itself and gets stuck in different ways. We have become accustomed to living our lives in a state of reactive stress—to the point that many of us aren't even consciously aware of when we're experiencing it anymore.

This section will show indicators of stress as they appear in each power center, how they impact you, and what variety of

stress is held there. Once we understand this, we build the awareness necessary to identify reactive stress and harness its energy
for motivation.

Movement Medicine and Breathwork

While the movement exercises in this book will help you flush
toxins, decrease bloating and inflammation, improve muscle
tone, and gain flexibility, their ultimate aim is to get to the root of
any discomfort and connect your mind, body, and heart.

When we are in our heads and out of our sensory bodies, we
are largely unaware of what is happening within us. We only
notice physical issues at the point where they have progressed
into a more serious problem. We come into our bodies by feeling
and slowing down to listen. The medicine of movement allows us
to move energy through our systems and enhance our physical
wellness by becoming more aware of our own presence.

When we are in touch with our bodies, we will know immediately when something is "off," and we can address smaller issues
before they become larger ones. Aside from that, we can continue
to work toward feeling even better.

It doesn't stop there. When we come into our body, we come
into so many other things as well. We come into our power, our
heart, our sense of inner knowing. When we come into our body,
we connect to our emotions and to clarity in our mind, but in
a different way than we do when we overthink and rationalize.
That nebulous mind-body connection we talk about so much?

This is it. And the movement exercises in this book combined
with a shift in mindset will get you there.

Throughout the course of this book, we'll use a lot of targeted breathwork. It is said that how we breathe is how we live. We want to breathe deeply, just as we want to live deeply. A superficial life might be easier sometimes, but is that really what you want at the end of the day?

Our breath brings us into our body, but it also connects us with our emotions. Through our breath, we become more present. We shift our attention from what we're doing next to *being* in the present moment. Our breath empowers us on a moment-by-moment basis.

In each power center, you will find a specific type of breathwork that speaks specifically to what we are aiming to accomplish in that area. Of all the exercises you will find in this book, the breathwork might just be the most powerful and transformative because you can use it at literally any time, in any situation, to transform your state almost immediately.

Heal and Rebalance

The ultimate goal with all of this is alignment. We are striving to align our body and, through that, to align our lives. With this aligned body comes greater body enjoyment and confidence, a deeper connection to true foundational strength and power, and a greater ease of movement through every step of life.

This doesn't have to be a chore. In fact, it can even be liberating, enjoyable, nurturing, relaxing, and super-restorative.

I will offer you a series of lifestyle tips that will facilitate healing, rebalancing, and reconnecting with a profound sense of joy: these tips range from turning up your favorite song and rocking out to taking in some fresh air to manifesting your ideal partner. What I love about all of these practices is that they can be easily incorporated into your daily life. Not only that, they will *enhance* your daily life in very real, measurable ways.

I recently discovered the power of healing baths while visiting a Korean spa. When I first looked at their herbal infusion, I wasn't sold. I decided to try it anyway, and I'm so glad I did. I emerged from the bath feeling renewed and reinvigorated, and my skin had a new glow to it. Each lifestyle section will end with a special bath designed to soothe, heal, and rebalance a specific power center. That's right—in each chapter, I'm going to recommend a bath with a special blend of herbs and salts. You don't need to do one every single night in order to feel the results, but I hope that you'll give them a try—the ritual, the moments of presence and peace, and the opportunity to focus on your body in a new way provide an enormous amount of comfort, cleansing, and healing.

Of course, baths cleanse us on a physical level, but they also cleanse us on an energetic level. The addition of salts and herbs can clear any energy that we pick up while going about our daily life, whether from our interactions with others or simply being in a world that can sometimes be petty and toxic. It's for this reason that going for a swim in the salty ocean is so cleansing.

Each chapter will also include aromatherapy, teas, herbs, crystals, and other soothing practices that you can experiment with. As I've said, not everything will resonate with everybody, but the goal here is to take you outside of your comfort zone and help you engage more deeply with parts of your body that deserve attention and care.

Part of taking care of ourselves is carving out a bit of "me time"—something we're all guilty of letting slide. The practices in this section will allow you to do that, whether you have a minute or an hour.

Visualization

Each chapter will end with a mantra and visualization. The visualizations here are likely different than any you've done in a meditation or yoga class, because they are very body-focused. Remember, the overarching goal of this book is for you to come *into* your body, not to leave it. With this in mind, we will work on grounding into and attuning with ourselves.

These visualizations can be done in a number of ways. You can mindfully read through them, conjuring up mental images as you go. You can record yourself reading the visualization aloud as a way of making it your own, then use it as a guided meditation. Or you can go to www.laurenroxburgh.com to download a free guided visualization as an accompaniment to this book.

Activate Your Superpowers

Each area of the body offers its own unique connection to a new resource of energy, connection, and deep strength. And each governs a certain quality that allows us to live life in a freer, more fully realized and empowered manner. When we are aligned and create space in that area of the body, we can bring the superpower into its fullest state.

Our pelvic floor awakens in us the sense of personal power

necessary to trust ourselves and move through the world with more grace and ease. Within our deep core, we find our connection to sensuality, which draws us more deeply into the experience of life. Our upper core provides us with the confidence to help us live our best life as our most authentic selves. Our heart allows us to nurture ourselves and give and receive love. And our head allows us to connect with wisdom that comes from a source greater than ourselves.

In the coming pages, we'll discuss all of these superpowers that dwell within us and begin to imagine what life might look like when we bring them into their most realized form.

Foods That Heal

While a balanced diet is crucial for holistic health, each power center has an affinity for specific foods. Interestingly, there is also an alignment between the color group of foods the power center needs to flourish and the color of the chakra associated with that power center. For example, the heart chakra is related to the color green, and the heart thrives with lots of leafy green vegetables. Incorporate these foods into your meals when you're looking for an extra boost or to give a certain power center a little bit of extra love and support.

Each chapter will include a selection of elixir, tonic, and broth recipes designed to bolster that specific power center. Elixirs, tonics, and broths offer us an efficient way to infuse healing minerals and nutrients into our diet. The recipes included are no-fuss and take a minimal amount of prep time. Many of them incorporate the herbs and superfoods that heal to make your restorative alignment regimen that much easier.

As I will discuss in the coming pages, I find both selecting and preparing food to be a nourishing practice of love—it is a daily way in which I show love to myself and to my family. As you prepare these foods, think of what you are really doing: nourishing your body and your energy, and providing yourself and those you love with life force. Viewed through this lens, preparing and enjoying food can be one of the most highly beneficial meditative practices available to us.

Putting It All Together

I have intentionally provided a wide variety of information and practices in this book to help empower you with knowledge, align your body, awaken your senses, connect you to the present, and find freedom in mind, body, and heart. More than likely, you will be drawn to certain practices more than others—this is great! Indulge in what moves and resonates with you the most.

I also challenge you to spend some time with those exercises that you feel more averse or resistant to. There's probably a reason for that as well. Give it a try, and you might just be surprised to find what opens up for you.

3

The Pelvic Floor Power Center: The Awakening Superpower

SIGNS YOUR PELVIC FLOOR NEEDS SOME LOVE

Physical

* Entire body constantly feels tight and tense
* Lower back pain
* A pooched lower belly
* Inability to connect with your core
* Pain during sex
* Leaking urine when exercising, laughing, coughing, or sneezing
* Difficulty orgasming

Emotional

* Needs are not met to the point where you can live comfortably
* Weak financial foundation
* Lack of support at home
* Fears that you and your family will not be okay
* Not feeling grounded

The Imbalanced Pelvic Floor

When Ellie came to me, she was feeling pretty despondent. Over the course of the past several years, she had given birth to three children. She felt as if her body had never fully recovered. Ellie's body was stuck in a state of clutch, and she constantly experienced lower back pain and thick, tight hips. Her pelvis was stuck in an anterior tilt (in other words, she had an arched spine), she was carrying extra weight, and she had a pooched belly. No matter how much she tried to conquer her belly with cardio work, Ellie couldn't get her core to activate. And these were just the physical symptoms! Ellie was also unable to stir up any sexual desire for her husband and was constantly weighed down with stress about her family and finances.

To say the least, Ellie wasn't enjoying her body or life. She had become a victim of stress, both physical and emotional.

I could immediately tell that Ellie was clutching, both figuratively and literally. Emotionally, Ellie was desperately clutching to the idea of getting healthy and looking and feeling good. Before coming to me, Ellie had already seen several doctors, trainers, bodyworkers, and physical therapists, none of whom had been able to help her. She tried everything, and yet nothing was working. In fact, things were getting worse. Ellie had some medical testing done before she came to me, and it was discovered that she was suffering from osteoporosis, had gained excess body fat, and had shrunk an inch in height. Because she couldn't activate her core, Ellie's muscles were atrophied and weak, and other areas of her body were compensating. It had gotten to the point where Ellie's neuromuscular connection was impeded—in other words, her brain and body were having a difficult time communicating. For this reason, she was experiencing lower back pain, weight gain, and general inflexibility.

As soon as I met Ellie, I could tell she was experiencing pelvic floor issues. She walked tightly and without a lot of graceful movement—there was no sway to her step at all, and a lot of rigidity in her joints. Because I specialize in the pelvic floor, it was clear to me that Ellie was clutching there, and that this was probably at the root of her issues. Yet none of the specialists Ellie had seen so far had so much as mentioned her pelvic floor.

As Ellie and I began working together, it became clear to me that she was predisposed to pelvic floor issues. The issues Ellie was currently experiencing would have arisen sooner or later, one way or the other, but the pregnancies made her more susceptible to them more quickly. This was aggravated by the fact that Ellie was constantly clutching her pelvic floor in reaction to stress. Because Ellie was feeling incredibly disempowered on many levels, she had been trying to exert power over her life through an almost aggressive attitude of attempting to control everything—her body, her stress, her family, their finances. She was clutching in every way. Ellie had lost her ability to feel the messages her body was sending her to surrender, allow, receive, and make herself a priority. Many people live their lives in this state—particularly mothers.

The first order of business was to teach Ellie how to connect with and awaken her pelvic floor. She had to understand that she was clutching before she could release it, so awareness and connection were key. Through a series of relaxation and activation movements and visualizations, which I will share below in this chapter, we gradually began to create a new brain-body connection for Ellie. This new connection was established by rewiring the nervous system, which carries messages from the brain down to the pelvic floor and vice versa. This reawakened muscles Ellie needed to target and reignited connections that were dormant.

Once Ellie was able to connect with her pelvic floor and feel the power there, I was able to teach her how to turn on and off that stress button we discussed in Chapter 1. Now, instead of *reacting* to the stresses of life, Ellie was becoming aware and taking empowered action.

Through this release and resiliency, Ellie was able to relax and let go of the heaviness and rigid energy that come from trying to force and control things that were beyond her control. She was able to more easily go with the flow of life.

I see many of my clients have the same realization Ellie experienced: we cannot control most of the circumstances of our life, but we *can* control how we react to them. Once she let go of the need to forcefully control everything, Ellie was able to navigate life and her body in a much more empowered way. She was able to activate her pelvic floor and find happiness and joy again. She was able to connect to an authentic confidence and enjoy the present moment with her beautiful family, rather than just fretting about them.

Very quickly, Ellie experienced relief on every level. The physical release of clutching relieved her of her back pain. She found a renewed lightness, deep abdominal connection, and flexibility. Because she was able to connect with her pelvic floor, Ellie's lower back and hips didn't have to compensate anymore, her hips became more fluid, and her pelvis came back into alignment, including the alleviation of that anterior tilt and reduction of the lower belly pooch she had been experiencing.

After we worked together for a few months, Ellie was retested. She found that her osteoporosis was gone, and she had lost 10 percent of her body fat and gained 1.5 inches in height. She stood up straighter and moved more gracefully and with more fluidity. She even wanted to have sex with her husband again! Needless to say, her doctor was floored and wanted to know how she did it.

Through all of this, Ellie discovered a new level of deep strength and personal empowerment. She began to trust her body, her instincts, and her ability to navigate life without trying to control it. She was able to reframe the stressors in her life as lessons to learn and grow from, rather than obstacles she had to plow through. She came to see the positive in nearly every situation. The same grace, resilience, and flexibility Ellie found in her body was also reflected in her life.

Get to Know Your Pelvic Floor

As a culture, the only time we really talk about the pelvic floor is when the topic turns to sex or pregnancy. This is a travesty, because this powerful area of our body offers us a wealth of strength, sensation, information, connection, and vitality that extends far beyond sex.

Not only do we rarely discuss all that the pelvic floor offers us, we don't even have a vocabulary to discuss what happens when things are not right. We talk openly about injuries or pain that we sustain in other parts of the body, but most people shy away from an open discourse when something goes wrong "down there." It's almost like we're embarrassed about this part of our body and the problems that arise when it isn't healthy. But as we've discussed, the pelvic floor impacts so many important bodily functions! Ignoring it might manifest into problems such as incontinence, pain during sex, inability to achieve orgasm, or more general pain that is usually the result of tightness. It can also present itself as tight hamstrings, a weak deep core and butt, a pooched belly, a hernia, lower back pain, impotence, or premature ejaculation. As we discussed in Chapter 1, most of us tend to clutch our pelvic floor. Just like a clenched fist cannot grasp, a too-tight pelvic floor is unable to support the proper positioning and optimal function of the pelvic organs, bones, and vertebrae.

The pelvic floor is architecturally fascinating and brilliantly designed. It consists of three layers of sixteen individual muscles, some of which are very small. These layers attach like a hammock to three points: the pubic bone, tailbone, and sitz bones. Our pelvic floor serves as the base of our deepest core, supports our organs, and, for women, supports our children when they are in utero. This hammock-like design is meant to ensure the pelvic floor can move and expand tremendously, contract powerfully, and release entirely. When we clutch the pelvic floor, we are thrown into an unnatural state of limited movement. The layers of tissue within the pelvic floor become glued down and fixed into a position that reinforces this unnatural constant contraction. Not only does this result in pain and dis-ease in the pelvic floor, but it also forces the rest of our body to compensate for it in a number of ways, which we will discuss throughout this book.

All of this means that, while we tend to associate pelvic issues with postpartum conditions (which they can be), they are issues that potentially impact all of us, whether we've had children or not, and whether we are female or male (although pelvic floor issues are more prominent in females, affecting up to one-third of all women in America). Over-stressing, over-training, overdoing, and sexual trauma can result in pelvic floor issues. So can sitting too much, which puts most of us in danger. If we were to counteract all of the time we spend sitting by moving, unwinding, meditating, and relaxing, our pelvic floor could remain healthy despite all of the time spent sitting. For most of us, though, this is not the case.

When we clutch our pelvic floor, its hammock-like base pulls in and up like a rosebud. While we do want the ability to clutch this area sometimes, it's important that it also has the ability and space to expand and bloom like a flower as well. Some people are in such a subconscious habit of clutching that they never allow this expansion to happen. It's a lot like when you clench your jaw too tightly—eventually, it begins to feel as if it's almost locked and glued in to a clenched position. This is uncomfortable at best, painful at worst, and not how the jaw was meant to function. Same with the pelvic floor—and they are deeply intertwined. The problem is, clutching is much easier to identify in the jaw than it is the pelvic floor because many of us are so disconnected from our pelvis.

This results in a hypertonic state, which means the pelvic floor becomes numb and weak, and loses its nerve connection. All of this tightness also impedes the flow of chi, which is particularly detrimental in the pelvic floor. Because our life force begins here, a blockage in the pelvic floor means that chi is also blocked in every other area of the body as well.

With tightness and a lack of connection also comes rigidity, weakness, disconnection, and pain. The pain is a result of your body desperately trying to communicate with you that a particular area needs some attention, space, movement, or change. While pain presents for this reason in all areas of the body, what makes the pelvic floor unique is that we're often not even aware of the pain. We've long since learned to live with it. Most of us have been unconsciously clutching the pelvic floor so consistently, and for so long, that we're not even aware we're stuck in an unnaturally frozen and weakened state. We are totally unaware of what comfort, relaxation, flexibility, and expansion even feel like in this area of the body. This clutched state has become status quo, and we are none the wiser.

Because the pelvis is an area of such connectivity, when you build resiliency in your pelvis by learning how to contract and relax your pelvic floor, you also release your hamstrings, inner thighs, sacrum, lower back, and hip flexors, while also helping reawaken your deepest foundational core muscles. *Ah*, freedom from those aches and pains that plague so many of us in our lower back and hip flexors! As if that's not enough, a relaxed, flexible, more connected and confident pelvis also makes sex more pleasurable, and in many cases climax easier to achieve. In fact, I have plenty of female clients who had a difficult time reaching orgasm—or never orgasmed at all—until they learned to awaken and relax their pelvic floor. Building this awareness and connecting to their pelvic floor completely transformed their ability to feel, be present, enjoy their own bodies, connect with their partners, and engage in deeper and more fulfilling intimacy and connection.

That's only the beginning. The health of our pelvic floor

directly impacts pretty much every area of our body and our life. This is why the topic is worthy of an entire book!

We're so trained to be in clutch that many of us don't know how to let go. I can't even begin to count how many clients I've had who have no idea what a pelvic floor is—and have even asked if men have one—let alone how to release it. They literally have no connection to this area of their body. If you find you have this same experience, rest assured, you're not alone. We want to resolve it, though, because when people are disconnected from their pelvic floor, it usually means that they are in a constant state of clutch and tension. This both results in and is indicative of a fear-based life. We clutch because we are struggling to survive. Or, at least, that's what our body is telling us.

Here's the good news: through my clients, I've also seen that once this issue is identified, it takes no more than a minute to walk through and create that connection between your brain and your pelvic floor to arouse a whole part of you that has been repressed for many years.

RESTORE YOUR PELVIC FLOOR

Once you learn to isolate the muscles of your pelvic floor in order to activate and relax them, you have the power to control how you deal with stress. When you clutch, you are indicating to your body and brain that you are stressed, compressed, and coiling in. When you relax your pelvic floor muscles, the rest of your body believes it and follows suit.

The following practice will empower you to understand how your body deals with stress, and where and how you hold stress. It will help you feel relaxed, calm, and strong, which can make you look and feel more vibrant and youthful. It will also help create more fluidity and flexibility in your hips and pelvis, and connect you to the base of your core.

Close your eyes and visualize the muscles at the base of your core, between your sitz bones, that you would use to cut your pee off midstream. Without using your tush or abs, contract your rosebud, pull it up and into your body, and hold it. You should feel a tightening around your vagina.

Contrast this move by letting go of the muscles, feeling space between your sitz bones, and allowing your rose to bloom. Feel the base of your core relax, and then relax and expand a little more from there until you experience a complete surrender of holding. You will feel your belly relax, your shoulders melt, and your jaw and head release. Do this in a series of 6 to 8 repetitions, anytime and anywhere. It might be while you are in the car, waiting in line, or even right before you meditate or do a workout to ignite your superpower.

At first, you will have to focus on maintaining this connection by reminding yourself to release over and over again. But the more you do it, the easier it gets, because you are building a brain-body, neuromuscular connection. Once you've made that connection and experienced the sensation (and benefits!) of intentionally releasing the pelvic floor, it becomes easier and easier to do.

I, too, used to totally lack this connection. And I lacked it even as a strong, competitive athlete who was generally very aware of my body. Still, I didn't have the slightest clue that I was in a constant state of clutching my pelvic floor. Generally speaking, I was more or less completely unaware of my pelvic floor and the magical powers it holds. The rigidity I held in my pelvic floor showed up in the inflexibility of my hamstrings and hips, super-tight jaw, the pain in my lower back, and my furrowed brow.

Like me, over time, you will be amazed to see what a big difference finding this release makes, not only on a physical level, but also on holistic and emotional levels.

The Hips

Our hips are also included in this power center. From a physical standpoint, the hips include a lot of attachments—muscles attach to bones, and bones attach to the hip joint. There are layers upon layers of connection in the hips, which serve the very important purpose of attaching our legs to our pelvis. It's important to be aware of this, because congestion is more likely in areas of attachment. The hips are a prime spot for this. Our hips were designed to move—that's precisely what all of these attachments are meant to facilitate.

You've heard the phrase "use it or lose it," right? That applies to the hips. When we spend too much time sitting or otherwise don't move the hips as we are meant to, all of these attachments and tissues become compressed, tight, heavy, and dense. We aren't extending, expanding, decompressing, stretching, or opening the hips as much as our bodies need to in order to thrive. It is a general rule of thumb that when we're not moving an area of our body, it becomes sluggish, thicker, denser, and weaker, and functions in a less-than-optimal way. In the modern world, our hips are particularly prone to lack of use, at least to the extent they were meant to be.

When our hips tighten, it actually shortens the length of our legs, and our hips grow wider and more compressed. We begin to walk with stiff, shortened, jerky steps rather than the graceful, fluid movements our hips are meant to facilitate. Without this fluid movement, we are not freeing up energy, flushing fluids, detoxifying, or releasing tension and emotions. We begin to experience knee and back pain as well as bad posture, which can bring our entire body out of alignment.

The Pelvic Floor and Holistic Health

Perhaps more than any other power center, the health of the pelvic floor impacts our overall holistic health. In Eastern traditions, the pelvic floor is believed to be the root or base from which we draw our life force energy, or chi. Just like a tree with lifted roots becomes unstable, such is the case with our bodies when our pelvic floor is out of alignment. If our pelvic floor is not properly connected and we don't feel rooted, connected, or grounded, it becomes impossible to balance and integrate the rest of the physical body and energetic system.

If you've been to a yoga class, at some point you've probably heard that we hold emotion in our hips. The experience of crying during hip-opening movements is actually quite common— maybe you've even experienced it yourself, like I did the first time I practiced yoga back in college.

When we open and relax our hips, we release the emotions stored there. Just as our hips can become congested physically, they can also become congested energetically and emotionally.

When we aren't processing or working through our emotions, they become stagnant, heavy, and stuck. We often experience this backlog in our hips, because they are so dense with all of the anatomical intersections that connect the upper body to the lower body. Whereas certain areas of the body are associated with specific emotions, the hips work in a more general sense. Any and all emotions can become stuck and lodged here. From an Eastern perspective, it is this blockage that stagnates our life force.

The Root Chakra

The root chakra, which is the first chakra, is located in the pelvic region and is associated with our reproductive glands. It is signified by the color red. This is where we store information about our primal foundation, or where we come from. It is the place from which both life and life force emanate.

It is believed that we store our family's wounds in our root chakra. In other words, some of our ancestors' pain and past experience still lives within us and manifests itself in our own lives. Eastern religions and philosophies look at this in a number of different ways. Hindu philosophies, for example, frame it as *pitra dosh*. This is believed to be a karmic debt of our ancestors that the living carry forth within their horoscope.

Maybe chakras aren't your jam, but epigenetics points to this same phenomenon through the Western lens of science. Epigenetics studies the way our genes express our heredity in ways that are not related to changes in the underlying structure of DNA. One of the most well-known examples of epigenetics at work is based on a study conducted by McGill University and

Douglas Mental Health University Institute. They learned that the children of women who were pregnant during a massive ice storm in Quebec showed distinctive DNA patterns based on their mothers' exposure to stress.

In other words, if your mother undergoes some type of trauma, it may be transferred to you on a genetic level. You may not ever be aware of this; however, if something traumatic happens in your own life, your reaction to it may be impacted by your genetic link to your mother's trauma. For example, you may be predisposed to panic attacks because that is how your mother's trauma impacted her. However, it's also important to know that this doesn't mean you're doomed to have panic attacks of your own. All of us are predisposed to certain conditions based on our heredity, but our lifestyle choices and mindset have been scientifically proven to trump genetic predispositions.

Researchers have recently found that chronic exposure to the stress hormone cortisol caused visible mutations in mice, which gave them a predisposition to stress. What this means for us is that if you were exposed to an excess of cortisol in utero, you may have undergone a cellular mutation that was transferred to you and predisposes you to stress.

This does not mean that your future is written in stone (or in your cells), but it does mean that you will want to take more preventative lifestyle measures to guard against stress than a person without this predisposition. The good news is that, in this specific example of inherited stress, lifestyle decisions and emotional hygiene constitute 95 percent of the cure. Rest assured, your fate is firmly in your control.

The Pelvic Floor and Stress

As we've already discussed, the vast majority of us are completely unaware that our pelvic floor lives in a constant state of clutch. When we are in clutch, we are either consciously or subconsciously stressed. Strengthening your pelvic floor is no small matter. If you're constantly clutching, you're chronically stressed, whether you realize it or not. Your nervous system is living in a state of stress. This stress manifests itself physically, as well, through issues like peeing when you laugh or sneeze; a tucked-under tailbone; a saggy tush; straining during bowel movements; weak hip rotators; and an overworked, sometimes painful lower back. These problems are all the result of clutching and a lack of energy flow—in other words, stress.

Remember those stuck emotions we discussed in the hips? This has a huge impact on our stress levels as well, because whenever emotion can't rise up and release, that energy gets stuck in the body and festers, creating dis-ease. That may present itself through literal sickness (because stress lowers our immunity) or through a more generalized and chronic feeling of stress.

Throughout this book, we will discuss lots of practical tools for reducing stress and nipping it in the bud on the ground floor—the pelvic floor.

PELVIC FLOOR STRESS HYGIENE

To begin building new, nonreactive habits around stress, try this simple stress-combating exercise the next time you catch yourself in a moment of clutching.

Gently ground your feet down into the earth, feeling your pinky toe, big toe, and heel, which I like to refer to as the tripod. Feel the ground under you and how the earth supports you. Allow yourself to experience a sense of presence and repeat, "I am safe," three times.

Movement Medicine for the Pelvic Floor

Creating space and strength in the pelvic floor, hamstrings, hips, and lower pelvis will connect you to a hidden part of your body that will help awaken a reconnection to a deep strength. This will offer a sense of support that you may not have felt for a long time. The pelvic floor is neglected in most movement modalities and even in most physical therapy or bodywork. Once you stimulate this part of your body, you will find a new source of energy. Through these movements, you will learn how to harness this energy for connection, creativity, motivation, and focus.

While these exercises call for a squishy ball, you can use any type of soft ball, such as a children's bouncy ball. If you would like to purchase my signature Body Sphere for these exercises, or to see my videos using the Sphere, please visit www.laurenrox burgh.com.

Safety note: Please start with a softer ball or Body Sphere for these exercises and work your way to a firmer version. Filling it up about 60–70 percent is perfect. If you already have a ball that is too full and too firm, then be sure to let some air out before doing these moves.

Sacred Space Sit

Come to a sitting position on the floor or your yoga mat. Place your squishy ball on the mat and bring your sitz bones down on the ball, crossing your legs. Allow your pelvic floor to expand over the ball and, using your hand, pull each sitz bone over the ball to allow the hammock of your floor to expand. Take a big inhale, and then exhale as you feel yourself grounding down into the ball and the earth. Next close your eyes to connect and take another inhale for a count of 8 and feel your diaphragm press down into your organs and expand your pelvic floor. On your next exhale, close your eyes and pull your pelvic floor up and into your body like a rosebud coiling up and in and hold for a count of 10. Then inhale for 8, soften your pelvic floor, and visualize that rosebud blooming as you sink down into the squishy ball, releasing stress and tension through the entire body. Repeat this movement 8 to 10 times.

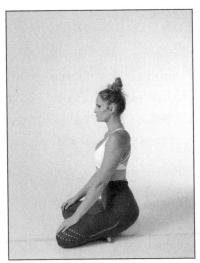 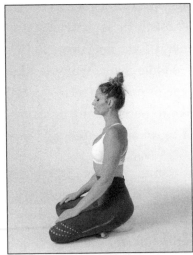

Sacred Space Sit

Seated Flex and Extend

Come to a sitting position on the floor or your yoga mat, place the squishy ball under your sitz bones, and cross your legs, allowing your pelvic floor to soften over the ball. Place your hands and fingertips on the edge of each knee. Inhale for a count of 8 as you extend and arch your spine, lift your heart, and look up. Then exhale for a count of 10 as you curl your tail under and bow your nose toward your pubic bone, while the ball rolls slightly forward. Repeat this series of movements 8 to 10 times.

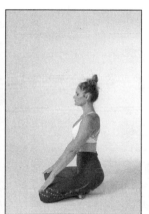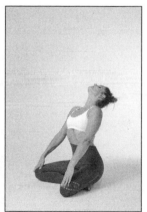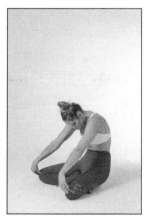

Seated Flex and Extend

Upright Spine Circles

Come to a sitting position on the floor or your mat. Place your squishy ball under you so that you are sitting on the ball, relaxing your sitz bones over the ball. Place your palms on your inner knees and gently press down to sit up tall. Inhale as you lean your upper body to the right. Exhale as you circle your torso forward over the mat. Inhale as you circle your body up to the left. Exhale as you lift your heart and spine back up to sit tall. Reverse the direction and repeat. Repeat this series of movements 8 to 10 times.

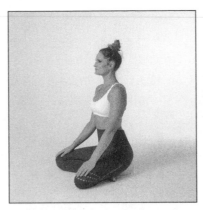
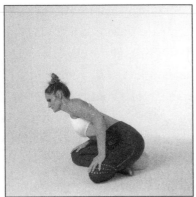
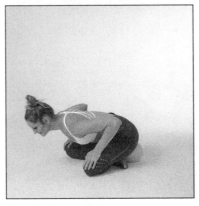
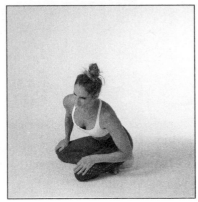

Upright Spine Circles

Hamstring Extension

Come to a sitting position on the floor or mat and place the squishy ball under your left sitz bones. Bend your right knee and place your right foot on the ground. Reach your arms a few inches back and place your fingertips down, facing out to the side.

Inhale as you open your heart and sit up tall. Then exhale as you roll your hips back, while the ball rolls down your left hamstring. Inhale as you roll back up to your sitz bone and come up to a tall spine. Repeat this series of movements 8 to 10 times.

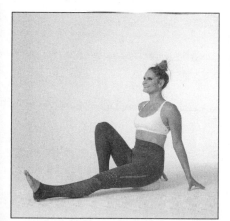
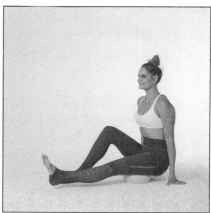

Hamstring Extension

Wide Lateral Split with Rotations

Come to a sitting position on your yoga mat. Place the squishy ball under your sitz bones. Extend both legs wide into a lateral split, leaving your knees slightly and softly bent. Reach your arms back, pressing your fingertips onto the mat behind you. Inhale, press into your fingertips, extend your spine, lift your heart, and flex your feet, reaching your toes up, while you rotate your sitz bones back and stretch your pelvis, inner thighs, ankles, and feet. Next, exhale as you internally rotate your legs and feet inward and point your toes down. Then rotate back out and circle the ankles out around and back up. Repeat this series of movements 8 to 10 times.

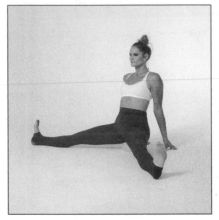

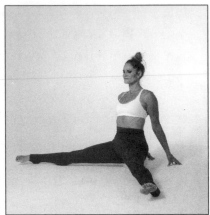

Wide Lateral Split with Rotations

Single Leg Split with Side Bend

Come to a sitting position on your yoga mat. Bring the squishy ball under you so that you are sitting on it, bend your left knee out to the side, and bring your left heel up against the ball. Extend your right leg out long to the right. Inhale and feel your pelvis drop down into the ball. Exhale and allow your tissues to soften. Inhale as you reach your left arm up. Exhale as you side bend over to the right, sliding your right hand along your

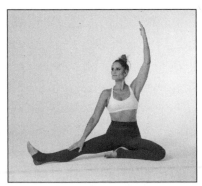

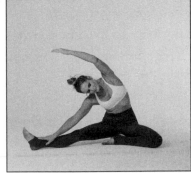

Single Leg Split with Side Bend

right shin. Inhale to come up. Repeat this series of movements 8 to 10 times.

Hip Flush

Sit on your yoga mat and place the squishy ball under your right hip. Extend your right leg long. Cross your left leg in front of you, placing your left foot on the mat. Place your right hand under your right shoulder. Inhale and bend your right knee to roll up the hip area. Exhale as you flush and roll down the hip. Repeat this series of movements 8 times on each side.

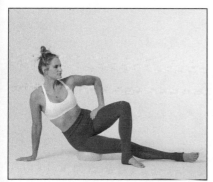 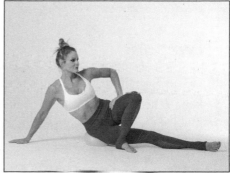

Hip Flush

Lower Back Massage

Come on to your side on your yoga mat and place the squishy ball under your right hip bone. Lower down onto your right forearm with your elbow underneath your shoulder. Place your right ankle on top of your left knee, with your left foot down on the mat, coming into a figure four position. Place your left hand on your right knee to further stretch and now inhale as you curl your tailbone up into a rounded lower spine. Next, roll and massage

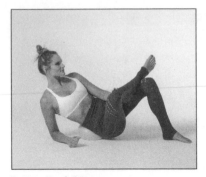 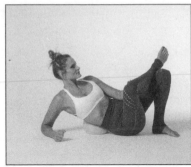

Lower Back Massage

your way back up the side of your lower back. Exhale as you roll down to the top of your hip, slightly arching your spine. Repeat this series of movement 8 to 10 times on each side.

Deep Squat

Come down in to a deep squat position on your yoga mat. Place the ball in the center of your mat. Take your feet out slightly wider than hips-width distance and turn out your toes so that your heels are internally rotated in. Bend your knees wide as you come down into a

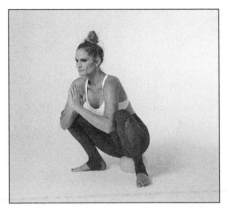 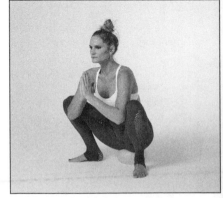

Deep Squat

deep squat to sit on the ball, bringing your hands into a prayer position. Inhale as you rock to the right, rolling the squishy ball to the left. Exhale as you roll to the left, rolling the ball to the right. Come back to center and ground into your feet, allowing your pelvis and pelvic floor to release. Repeat this series of movements 8 times.

Butterfly Split

Place the ball at the center of your yoga mat and sit on it, taking your knees out wide into a butterfly split, with your heels in toward your tush. Place the palms of your hands on your thighs. Inhale as you lean your torso to the left, while you press your right knee down with your right hand. Next, exhale as you lean to the right, pressing your left knee down with your left hand. Repeat this series of movements 8 to 10 times.

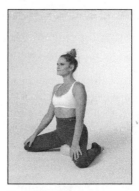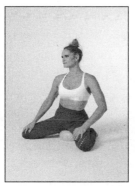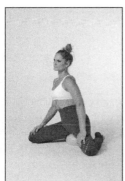

Butterfly Split

Breathe into Your Pelvic Floor

Come to a seated position on a chair or your yoga mat. We are going to practice expanding and contracting your diaphragm and pelvic floor as you breathe.

When you inhale, feel your lungs expand as the diaphragm moves down into your organs and pelvic floor, expanding the base of your core and releasing blocked energy and tension. As you exhale, feel the pelvic floor and diaphragm lift upward to close the ribs and flush and cleanse the lungs, bringing out the stagnant CO_2. Repeat this intentional breath 5 times, slowly filling all the way up with air as you inhale, then exhaling all of the air out.

Heal and Balance Your Pelvic Floor

Hang Out with Mother Nature

In Chinese medicine, there are four elements: earth, air, water, and fire. Different areas of the body are associated with each element. For example, our grounding chakra—the root chakra, a.k.a. our pelvic floor—is associated with the element of earth. Being around literal earth and roots helps balance this area of the body. When the pelvic floor is surrounded by earth energy, it is literally in its element.

This means that simply spending time with Mother Nature is healing for the pelvic floor and can help you connect with this area of your body. Make some time in your day—even if it's just a few minutes—to get out and experience the sounds and smells of nature. Turn your phone on airplane mode or, even better, leave it behind. Look at the trees and how their roots connect them to the earth. Feel the earth beneath you as you walk. Soak in the smell of the grass, trees, plants, and soil. Sit on the grass under a tree and physically connect your pelvic floor with the earth—zone out, feel your body, meditate, read a book, or have a picnic. What you do isn't as important as experiencing that physical connection to the earth.

Forest Bathing

There is a practice called "forest bathing" (or *shinrin-yoku*) in Japanese culture. In the early 1980s, the Forest Agency of Japan encouraged people to get out in nature; this was not about literally bathing in a forest—it was about basking in the lush richness of forests. Since then, scientific research has pointed to the fact that forest bathing improves mood and energy levels while reducing stress. It has also proven to lower heart rate and blood pressure and bolster immunity. Forest bathing doesn't involve major effort, like hiking—it involves just being, feeling, and soaking in. If you can't get to a forest, a park will do.

Get in Touch with the Cycles of the Earth

For women, the pelvic floor is all about cycles—after all, this is where we menstruate, which is sometimes known as a woman's "moon cycle." This is appropriately named, because our ovulation is influenced by the moon. (Did you know that peak rates of conception occur right around the full moon?) Each month, an egg ripens, and we either become pregnant or release the egg. This is an elemental cycle of creation. In many cultures, this cycle is viewed as sacred—which it absolutely is.

Gardening can be an extremely healing practice while bringing awareness to our own cycles, because gardening is all about cycles. Not only does gardening connect you with roots and Mother Nature, but it also aligns you with the natural cycles and rhythms of the earth and life. Gardening reminds us that, just like our gardens require something a little different each day to thrive, so too do our bodies.

Spend time in your garden, and if you don't already have one, consider planting one. It doesn't have to be big or complex; an indoor herb garden that you cultivate in a pot or a window box will suffice. In fact, maybe you just want to dedicate yourself to growing a single plant. Whatever you choose to do, be intentional as you care for it. Notice the roots, the scents, and how it grounds down into the earth; be aware of its various cycles and its fertility. Witness the power of creation through your garden.

Cook with Intention

We don't necessarily think of it this way, but food is the most basic and fundamental form of life force. Food sustains and nourishes us. As we've discussed, life force is always associated with the pelvic region, since our chi emanates from that area of our body. I love bearing this in mind as I go to the farmer's market and gather an abundance of fresh ingredients. I take my time carefully selecting the colors and flavors that will enliven and nourish my family. I bring them home with gratitude and cook with intention. I think about how I want to infuse my family with the love, healing, and life force that this food offers.

I also find cooking itself to be a meditative and grounding practice. We spend so much of our days in the masculine yang state of doing, and live in a yang "get-it-done" world. Cooking calls upon our healing and receiving yin energy, which means that it calls upon the feminine, creative, nurturing part of our nature—for women and men. In this yin state, we can relax, be present, and feel again. Gathering fresh ingredients from the earth, smelling the ingredients, tasting the food, cooking, sipping on a glass of wine, and sharing and breaking bread with your friends and family all help awaken your senses, calm your nervous system, and help bring you more into the present moment.

While you may not be able to prepare every meal in this manner, doing so for just one meal per week will bring some balance and grounding into your life. Don't worry about getting fancy or preparing multiple courses—if you're not comfortable in the kitchen, just start with something that feels simple and easy that allows you to engage with great ingredients and try new spices. You could even just start by preparing a salad with a rainbow assortment of different chopped vegetables! You can allow the practice of cooking to be a healing sanctuary of sorts.

Choose What You Bring into Your Life

You can emotionally shift the state of your physical pelvic floor and emotional roots by making intentional choices about who and what you surround yourself with and where and when you spend your time. What better way to enact power over your own life than by making conscious decisions about the energy you give and take in it?

I am including this as a lifestyle tip because we spend so much of our time making decisions—often subconsciously—about who and what we bring into our world. In fact, your entire life is a series of choices. Your relationships are a choice, how you spend your time is a choice, and who you spend your time with is a choice. Make a point of being aware of these decisions throughout your day. Seize your own power to surround yourself with what feels good to you.

TAKE A SEA SALT AND MUGWORT BATH

1 cup sea salt

12 ounces mugwort loose-leaf tea, brewed

For an overall tune-up, dissolve sea salt and mugwort into your bath. Mugwort, or *Artemisia vulgaris*, is known for its healing properties and calming effects. Mugwort is also used as a natural topical anesthetic with antibacterial and antifungal properties. When applied to the skin, it can help relieve burning, itching, and pain. It also helps alleviate eczema and skin irritations. Mugwort bath tea is simple to make at home. All you need is some dried, crushed mugwort leaves, which you can order on Amazon. To create tea, simply steep the mugwort leaves in hot water.

This bath is best taken right before bed because mugwort helps promote relaxation and deep, restorative sleep. In ancient cultures, mugwort was used as a uterine stimulant to bring on delayed menstruation and help restore a woman's natural monthly cycle.

To prepare this bath, draw your bath as usual. While the tub is filling, brew the mugwort tea. Use a strainer to capture the leaves and pour the tea into your bath. Loose-leaf mugwort tea can be found at your local health store or online.

Mantra and Visualization for the Pelvic Floor

"I am grounded, supported, and abundant."

Find a comfortable position, sitting on a cushion or a squishy ball. Cross your legs and feel your sitz bones become heavy. Now feel your spine line up in a neutral position. Shrug your shoulders up to your ears, take a big inhale, and exhale as they melt back down. Allow your entire body to relax.

Bring your attention to the anatomical structure in the base of your core, the beautiful hammock of strength, support, fluidity, and power. Now visualize that circular hammock of muscles drawing in and upward, like a rosebud. Pull it up and in to your organs and hold it, trying not to use any other muscles, including your upper abdominals and hip flexors. Slowly release the pelvic floor down, feeling the rose bloom. Notice how your whole spine, from your head to tail, softens into a surrender energy. Feel your entire nervous system begin to settle into a calm state.

Draw your pelvic muscles up again and notice the energy. This is the energy of control and making things happen. It is the energy of force. Soften your muscles and notice how your shoulders and jaw also melt. Notice your entire body connecting to a surrender energy. This is the nurturing, feminine energy of being, healing, and letting go.

This is the difference between control and letting go, between tension and softness. We need both of these energies at different points during life, not just to survive, but to thrive. When we deepen our awareness of these energies, we have a much deeper connection to ourselves, to our authentic paths, and to who we are and why we're here.

Bring the awareness again down low into your pelvic floor. Keep your energy in that soft surrender, noticing how there is a sense of calm, peace, and presence when you let go. That sense of presence is where happiness, joy, and connection to yourself and everyone and everything around you lies.

Stay in this light, easy energy, in the calm state of rest-and-digest, feeling the relaxation, the connection, and the groundedness of this energy in the base of your core. Feel how important it is for the rest of your spine and body. Notice how this calm energy actually helps you expand bigger, like a balloon. Your energy is no longer compressed down; now it can expand outwardly. Energetically, you can enjoy that beautiful, vibrant, glowing energy.

It all starts here.

Activate Your Awakening Superpower Through the Pelvic Floor

It is in the pelvic floor that we awaken our sense of empowerment by finding grounding and security in our lives. As we move up through the power centers, we will build upon this personal power, but first we must awaken it. We awaken our power at our very foundation—the pelvic floor.

When your pelvic floor is healthy and in balance, you feel secure in yourself, grounded in your life and in the world. Creation flows through you and your daily tasks feel effortless and in flow. You have a firm understanding of your place in the world, and a deep understanding of and alignment with what does and does not work for you in all aspects of your life. You learn to flow with the world rather than pushing against it.

The pelvic floor serves as our foundation and teaches us how to have balance in our bodies and lives. When our foundation is healthy, flexible, and functions well, we open up to our true, authentic power. Our roots are stable and fertile, which allows us to grow naturally and with ease. When we are grounded, we can rest in the comfort of feeling solid, strong, and calm.

If you're not there yet, that's okay. I think you'll be amazed to see how much easier it becomes to cultivate a sense of overall empowerment once you awaken this connection. From that point on, you will find freedom and empowerment—the sky is the limit in terms of true transformation and personal growth. However, we cannot grow, flow, and improve until we feel grounded, safe, and secure. To do this, we must expunge all of the physical clutching, ignite this dormant strength, and flush the retention of stagnant emotion and congestion that happens in this power center.

We previously discussed how, through intentional effort, we can create a greater connection between our brain and pelvic floor. This connection provides both physical and health benefits, but it also makes us feel more empowered in a more general sense.

Finally, a big part of how we express our personal power is through creation. Creation can look so many different ways, depending upon our unique gifts and talents. However, here in the pelvic floor, we hold the capacity for the greatest creative endeavor of all—the ability to create new life.

ALTERNATIVE THERAPIES FOR THE PELVIC FLOOR

Aromatherapy

Lavender and cedar are both very healing and balancing for the pelvic floor because they are earthy and calming scents. They encourage our senses to feel more grounded, calm, and stable. Since it is in the earth element, the root area where our stress center is located, you can see why these qualities are so effective and vital to our well-being.

Crystals

Throughout history, crystals and sacred stones have been used to clear, transform, and align energy and physical health. As otherworldly as it sounds, the cells of your body are made up of the same energy as healing crystals. Placing certain crystals over your body and in your environment helps the electromagnetic energy in your body awaken, transform, move, and align. Many believe that crystals can even harness energy from the quantum field to deliver it to your field of energy, kind of like a radio signal. Here are some of the crystals that are known to help clear, ground, and heal your pelvic floor.

- **Hematite**—absorbs toxic emotions and clears negative feelings of anxiety and worry
- **Red jasper**—grounds, stabilizes the mood, and soothes anxiety
- **Smoky quartz**—balances, grounds, and releases negative feelings of jealousy and anger

To heal your pelvic floor, select the crystal that resonates with you most and place it on your pelvic area. As it rests there, meditate, relax, or visualize the outcome you hope to receive. For a more consistent infusion of healing vibes, you can also carry your selected crystal with you in your purse or pocket, wear it as jewelry, or place it in your home or car.

I particularly like to place crystals in my bedroom so that I can receive their healing benefits while I sleep. This is a potent way to use crystals, because when we sleep our subconscious mind kicks into gear and deep healing occurs. Try placing the crystal either under your pillow or on the side of your bed. Take note of how your dreams are affected, and notice if you feel more rested the next morning.

Tea

Ginger tea is made from the roots of ginger plants. These roots grow deep within the earth. Based on its origins, this tea helps keep us grounded and embodies the energy of the root chakra.

Aside from that, ginger has some very practical purposes, including its ability to reduce inflammation and treat inflammatory conditions. It has also been found to reduce the symptoms of dysmenorrhea, the severe pain that some women experience during the menstrual cycle.

Of course you can buy bags of ginger tea, but it's easy to make as well. I like to chop up a knob of ginger, cut it up in small pieces, and steep it in water for 10 to 15 minutes. Strain before serving and enjoy!

Nourish Your Pelvic Floor

Herbs for the Pelvic Floor: Sage

Sage is known for its ability to clear energy. This is particularly important in the pelvic floor because we hold so much emotion—and, thus, stagnant energy—here. Also, since our pelvic floor marks one of the ends of our neuropathway, if we can clear the energy here, it will have the domino effect of clearing energy and releasing blockages throughout our entire system.

The great thing about sage is that it can be used in so many different forms. Of course, you can ingest it through teas and as a way of flavoring your food. You can also burn sage sticks and use them either to clear the energy in your space (home, office, etc.) or around yourself.

To use a sage stick to purify or cleanse your space (known as smudging), walk around the perimeter of the area holding your burning sage stick. Be sure to pay special attention to all of the corners and doorways. You want to focus on corners, because it is believed more energy tends to get stuck there. As for doorways, it is believed we tend to think a lot as we come in and out of doorways—about where we're going and where we've been—so they therefore hold more energy. If you notice that the smoke becomes grayer in a certain area, it is indicative that more stagnant energy is being held there.

You can also place sage on a ceramic tray and allow it to burn down. If you are going to smudge yourself, make sure that you do so outside so that you are releasing the energy rather than trapping it in your space.

Vitamins and Minerals for the Pelvic Floor

VITAMIN C

Vitamin C, or ascorbic acid, is a water-soluble vitamin that is essential for the growth, development, repair, and maintenance of several tissues and organs of the body. It also plays a crucial role in the synthesis of collagen, which is an essential component of the ligaments that hold the pelvic floor and pelvic organs.

I prefer to take Vitamin C in chewable tablets, or in powder form for maximum absorption.

CALCIUM

Calcium is the most abundant mineral in the human body. Apart from playing a major role in the contraction of the muscles and blood vessels, in hormone synthesis, and in central nervous system function, calcium also helps strengthen teeth and bones, including the pelvic bones.

Calcium is best absorbed in powder form in tandem with magnesium, because this is the most bioavailable form, which means the body can absorb it more efficiently. I prefer taking calcium in powdered form (which can be sourced easily on Amazon) and mixing it with water. Dark, leafy greens are also a great source of calcium.

IRON

Iron is important to supplement during our menstrual cycle to make up for blood loss. Additionally, iron deficiency affects up to 10 percent of women, and can present itself as fatigue and dizziness.

The best way to absorb iron is through food sources, such as grass-fed beef and green, leafy vegetables.

FOODS THAT HEAL THE PELVIC FLOOR

- **Root vegetables**—beets, carrots, garlic, ginger, onions, parsnips, potatoes, and radishes
- **Protein-rich foods**—beans, eggs, meats, and nuts
- **Spices**—cayenne, chives, horseradish, hot paprika, and pepper
- **Red-colored foods**—red apples, red cabbage, and strawberries

Root-Rebalancing Tonic

MAKES 8 OUNCES

Many people haven't heard of the herb lady's mantle, but it is a powerful and balancing herb for women. It helps relieve menstrual aches and pains, can reduce—or even stop—spotting between periods, and can lessen menstrual bleeding. (For best results, drink this tonic in the week leading up to your period.) Lady's mantle also helps during menopause as a result of its anti-inflammatory properties. More specifically, women with pelvic organ prolapse may benefit from lady's mantle because it helps heal vaginal tissues and lifts the pelvic organs upward. You can find lady's mantle at a healthy grocer like Whole Foods, or online.

1 cup hot water
1 teaspoon lady's mantle herb
1 teaspoon lemon balm

Steep the lady's mantle and lemon balm in the hot water for about 7 minutes. Pour the liquid through a strainer and into a mug to enjoy.

The Goddess Elixir

MAKES 8 OUNCES

This elixir finds its foundation in the beet, which is a root. This makes it the perfect match for the root part of our body. The apple adds a little dash of sweetness.

In both Ayurvedic and Chinese medicine, root vegetables are believed to have a very grounding, earthly energy. In the yogic tradition, ginger is viewed as a spice that heals the root chakra. It also helps the pancreas metabolize sugar and stimulates digestion and elimination. If you don't have fresh ginger on hand, you can swap in 2 teaspoons of powdered ginger.

1 small beet, scrubbed and peeled
2 red apples, cored and chopped
½ inch fresh ginger

Place all the ingredients in the juicer and be ready to feel an earthly goddess energy come through your blood.

Root-Rejuvenating Bone Broth

MAKES 8 TO 10 BOWLS

The pelvic floor loves foods that help us feel grounded, cozy, and warm from the inside out. This recipe includes ingredients such as buckwheat that help deepen our connection to Mother Earth and keep our physical structure strong. This broth is nutrient-dense: it's packed with magnesium, glucosamine, calcium, silicon, and phosphorus. All of these nutrients are easy to digest and rich in flavor. The collagen found in high-quality bone broth such as this helps our bodies create healthier connective tissue, which is key for a healthy pelvic floor. The collagen also helps keep skin stay smooth and glowy and even reduces the appearance of cellulite and wrinkles.

2 tablespoons olive oil

2 leeks, sliced lengthwise and thinly

2 celery stalks, sliced (throw in a few chopped leaves too)

2 large carrots, peeled and diced

1 cup buckwheat (toasted or raw), rinsed

2 teaspoons thyme

2 teaspoons fennel seeds

32 ounces organic bone, vegetable, or mushroom broth

Juice of one lemon

Himalayan salt, to taste

Pepper, to taste

A few springs of parsley, to garnish

Capers, to garnish

Drizzle the olive oil in a large pot over medium heat. Add the leeks and celery and cook until they are soft, stirring occasionally, for around 4 to 5 minutes. Add the carrots and cook for another 4 minutes. Add in the buckwheat, thyme, fennel seeds, broth, lemon juice, and salt and pepper to taste. Bring the pot to a boil, then reduce the heat to low and simmer, partially covered, for 15 minutes.

Serve the soup hot with parsley and capers to garnish.

To store, allow the broth to cool to room temperature before refrigerating or freezing. Store in an airtight container in the refrigerator for 5 to 7 days or in the freezer for up to 4 months.

4

The Deep Core Power Center: Sensuality Superpower

SIGNS YOUR DEEP CORE NEEDS SOME LOVE

Physical

* Pain in your sacrum
* Slow digestion
* Bloated, thick, and heavy waist
* Disconnected to true appetite
* Carrying weight in your lower belly area
* Low immune system
* Constipated

Emotional

* Swallowing emotions
* Difficulty seeing things clearly
* Lack of imagination
* Self-loathing thoughts
* Disconnected from emotions
* Feeling separate and disconnected from others
* Feeling better than others
* Judgmental feelings toward self and others
* Overthinking and overprocessing
* Misalignment of thoughts, words, and actions
* Inability to keep promises
* Difficulty communicating feelings
* Lack of a feeling of connection with something bigger than yourself

The Imbalanced Deep Core

Donna came to me because she was experiencing chronic constipation, bloating, and a pooched-out belly. She couldn't button her
jeans. She couldn't tell if she was hungry or not, and hadn't felt butterflies in her belly in years. Donna was super stressed out because
of her relationship with her husband and other family-related
issues. She didn't feel good about herself, and the last thing she
wanted was to touch her husband or to be touched herself.

Once I learned that all of Donna's discomfort was coming from
her belly area, her issue was pretty easy to target. We focused on
bringing her awareness to the area where she was having the most
discomfort (her deep core) to give her some relief. We practiced
movement medicine, concentrating on massaging her organs, and
did a lot of breathwork. We worked on creating space between the
rib cage and hips, which gave her organs more room to move and
function in a healthy way so that she could detoxify, connect and
release emotions, and properly digest.

Before long, Donna's thickness, inflammation, and scar tissue
melted away. She released bloat and constipation. She could tell
when she was hungry and when she wasn't. Not only did Donna's
jeans fit, but they were loose. She didn't even lose any weight; it
was all a result of decreasing inflammation and congestion.

While her appearance changed significantly, most noteworthy
was how it changed the way in which Donna functioned. She began
tasting her food better, feeling her gut instincts again, and was
present as she nourished herself because she could feel how food
was making her feel. She started gardening, going to the farmer's
market, and really enjoying and interacting with the world around

her. Without her belly pooch, Donna felt sexier. It was as if the real Donna was being revealed, both physically and emotionally. As I've seen with many of my other clients, unlocking her deep core filled her with powerful and attractive energy—in every way.

Get to Know Your Deep Core

Imagine the rings inside of a tree; your core has layers in much the same way. Those layers consist of muscle, connective tissue, organs (including the female reproductive system), the digestive system, nerves, and lots of emotional energy. In the Western world, we tend to focus only on the muscle layer of our core, but all of these components are equally important, not only for our physical wellness but also for healing and restoring core muscles.

Your deep core is located around the belly button area. The core also includes the psoas, which is considered either a hip flexor or core muscle, depending upon your school of thought. I consider the psoas to be part of the core because, although it is connected to the hip flexors, it is located higher up in the body and connects our torso to our legs. The psoas attaches from behind the organs, in front of the spine, and right under the diaphragm. It runs all the way through the hips into the groin. If our psoas is tight and imbalanced, so are our organs and pelvis.

The psoas is a stabilizing, connective muscle. It is responsible for bringing our legs forward when we walk. Despite this, most people walk from the hip joint down because they are disconnected from their psoas and core. To determine whether you are walking from your psoas or from your hips, notice if your steps feel long and graceful (psoas) or short and heavy (hips). If you are channeling Gisele's dancer-like runway walk or LeBron's grace-ful swagger down the court, you are moving as you are meant to. Your steps should feel expansive, fluid, and flowing.

When we learn to use the psoas as it was intended, we can attain a flatter belly; more flexible hips; a longer, leaner, and stronger core and back; and a more streamlined waist. Utilizing our psoas changes our posture and helps undulate the spine while giving us length and expansion. When we connect with and uti-lize our psoas, we reorganize our entire core and create more space and support. This impacts not only how we stand and walk for the better, but also how we breathe.

In ancient society, the psoas was known as the muscle of the soul because it connects us to intuition or "gut feelings." Taoists believe the psoas connects us to our ancestry and that our emo-tions and fears can become trapped in its delicate tissue. When we release these fears, we can begin to live from a more intuitive, sensual place. By physically awakening and connecting with the psoas, we can release trapped emotions, deep tension, and fears, which allows us to tap into sensuality and intuition.

Finally, our adrenal glands live right above our kidneys in the deep core. When we exist in a constant state of adrenal fatigue or fight-or-flight, it's almost impossible to connect to our creative energy and powerful intuition. Intuition can exist only when we are in rest-and-digest mode. Without our intuition, it is almost impossible to connect to those things we want to authentically manifest.

This means that, in a very real way, the stress we hold in our deep core impacts not only our ability to accurately sense our instincts and intuition, but also to feel our purpose and follow our life path.

We talk about our "gut feelings," but few of us really appreciate the amazingly strong connections between the brain and the digestive system. The stomach and intestines actually have more nerve cells than the entire spinal cord, almost like a mini-brain. The vagus nerve, which connects our brain to our guttural nervous system, is also located in our deep core. Vagus means "wandering" in Latin. This is appropriate, because the vagus nerve branches out from the two stems that connect the abdomen to the cerebellum and brainstem, touching our heart and other major organs as it winds up the body. It acts as a highway, carrying information from the brain to the digestive system and vice versa.

When we get in touch with our core, we create space in our waist and also improve digestion and even become better attuned with hunger. I have had clients resolve chronic IBS and indigestion issues by working their psoas, because moving, releasing, and strengthening this area decreases compression and inflammation. We develop an innate understanding of what our body needs and can eat more intuitively. Tuning in and providing our body with the right nutrition can alleviate or even resolve any number of issues.

The Deep Core and Holistic Health

From a physical standpoint, our deep core impacts everything from digestion to mobility to the largest organ, our skin.

When we are in tune with our deep intrinsic core, we are able to release pain, shrink our waist, improve posture and digestion, and even connect with and express our emotions in a healthier, more fully realized way. We feel more youthful and energetic, and our mind is clearer. Our awareness, vitality, and sensuality are all heightened.

This heightened sensuality allows us to feel more alive and in tune with our path and purpose. When we acknowledge who we are and what we want, it becomes so much simpler to magnetize those things, experiences, and people we desire into our lives. Our inner compass is recalibrated, which serves us in several different ways. We have an innate understanding of who "our people" are, and are able to cultivate real connection and intimacy with them in a natural, comfortable way. This also impacts our physical health, because we gain the ability to sense when something is not quite right physically, whether it's a little glitch or a larger imbalance in the body.

The Sacral Chakra

The deep core is associated with our sacral chakra, which is located right above the belly button and associated with the color orange and the element of water. Physically, this chakra is associated with the adrenal glands, which regulate our immune system and metabolism. It also governs the sex organs, digestive organs, bladder, skin, and lower back. Emotionally, the sacral chakra rules our feelings, including our ability to feel passion and sensuality. It also governs self-worth and integrity. How we balance all of these elements is based on the well-being of our sacral chakra.

This chakra is also connected to our sense of taste and food. It makes sense that the two seemingly disparate areas of feelings and food would be governed by the same chakra. I'm guessing you can see in your own life how closely your eating habits and emotional state are related. When the sacral chakra is balanced, we eat to thrive rather than to fill a void.

An imbalanced sacral chakra can either result in a highly emotional state or an underemotional state. Either way, this imbalance makes it very difficult to express ourselves clearly. Imbalance can also present itself as getting lost in fantasies, excessive behavior or addiction, a lack of feeling fulfilled, codependent behavior, and even sometimes infertility.

The Deep Core and the Pelvic Floor

Clutching our pelvic floor impacts everything, but it has a direct impact on our deep core. Compression in the pelvic floor directly translates to compression in the organs, waist, and lower spinal discs, which all lead to a thicker belly and hips and more tension in the deep core.

When our pelvic floor is clutched, it locks down our organs, found in the deep core. Often, when my clients release their pelvic floor, they find they can eliminate more easily and have a flatter belly and a more hourglass waist. This is because, when the pelvic floor is released, the organs can drop down into the floor of the pelvis, where they are meant to live. A good sign that you're clenching your pelvic floor and, in turn, compressing your organs is when you have the appearance of a beer belly. We often assume this belly is an indicator that we need to shed a few pounds. If you are clutching your pelvic floor and your pelvis is misaligned, that overly pooched belly is often your inflamed organs that are squished and stagnant excess fluids that create the fluff.

When your organs are wound up and tight, digestion, elimination, and absorption of nutrients are all impeded. You will feel bloated, constipated, and experience a lack of connection to your hunger levels as a result. Many people experience this by never feeling full, no matter how much they eat.

You may have a difficult time losing weight, no matter how you change your diet. Aside from the position of your organs, this is also often because of bloat due to compression, inflammation, inefficient elimination, and holding on to excess water as a result. When we release the pelvic floor and dislodge the tension in the belly, many people say they feel lighter, more flexible, calmer, and more fluid. What they are actually referring to is feeling less bloated because of better elimination, a lymphatic fluid flush, and a release of water retention.

Compression, tension, and toxins in the belly can also lead to inflammation. Inflammation in this area of the body can destroy gut flora, the good bacteria that help combat viruses; aid in digestion; and enhance absorption in our intestinal track. It can also lead to the development of bad bacteria, which can negatively impact the ability to burn fat.

Coming back to the gut-brain connection, it's important to understand that, when inflammation occurs, it's not an issue that's confined to the gut or digestion. That inflammation has a direct line to the brain thanks to our old friend, the vagus nerve.

Inflammation can occur on the cellular level and impact our brain, which can result in anxiety and depression. Serotonin— the happy hormone—can be inhibited, which negatively impacts our mood. And if all of this isn't enough, it is now believed that this type of cellular inflammation may play a role in the development of ADHD and Alzheimer's.

When our organs are tied up, we also have more trouble

flushing toxins. This might present itself as pain, dull skin (or even skin issues like eczema), a muffin top, or cellulite.

Seventy percent of the cells that make up our immune system are also housed in the deep core, so if your organs and glands are compressed, your immune system may be impeded. You will be more susceptible to sickness. This doesn't just apply to things like the flu and common colds, but also chronic and even fatal diseases such as cancer. Our immune system isn't meant to be constantly fighting off illness and disease. It also rejuvenates us when we sleep. If our immune system is always fighting, fighting, fighting, fighting, we will feel exhausted and sluggish and it can't do the deep repair to maintain vitality.

The Deep Core and Stress

Stress causes an increase in the production of cortisol, the stress hormone. When we are under stress or pressure, we release cortisol. This reaction is an evolutionary throwback to our fight-or-flight response, which served a very important purpose in our survival in earlier days. Cortisol can still serve a purpose in modern life, but it becomes a problem when we are in a constant state of fight-or-flight and our cortisol levels run wild.

This cortisol surge is functional when you are driving and get cut off. That rush you feel helps you react quickly so that you don't get in an accident. However, we were designed to have these cortisol-pumping reactions in severe situations, such as being chased down by lions—not every time we get a notification on our phone.

When too much cortisol is surging through the body, we age

prematurely, we may lose our hair, our skin and connective tissues dry up, we become wrinkled and saggy, our eyes sink in and develop bags under them, and our nails get brittle. This seems like a high price to pay, but it's because it takes so much out of our body to produce this reaction. High levels of cortisol can result in weight gain that no amount of dieting, working out, or even fasting can resolve; an inability to sleep; and even fertility problems. Cortisol also influences inflammation. As we discussed in the previous section, inflammation causes a trickle-down effect of symptoms that are stressful in their own right. Thus, when inflammation presents itself due to stress, it often becomes a vicious cycle of other chronic symptoms and issues, which exacerbate that stress even more.

Breaking the stress reaction cycle is a tricky business. Later in the chapter, we'll talk about mental and physical exercises that can help, but one less-talked-about way to manage stress is to think about the level of acidity in the body. Achieving an alkaline state in the gut is very healing, both in terms of wellness and stress levels. The number one thing that makes us acidic is stress. So, regulating stress and raising alkalinity help alleviate inflammation, regulate cortisol, and balance out the adrenals. Today, many of us have an acidic pH level, which opens the doorway to disease, including cancer. We do need some acid in our body, but on average, we want to achieve a balance of 80 percent alkalinity, 20 percent acidity.

Determining your body's pH level is as easy as picking up a test at your local pharmacy or on Amazon. Simply urinate on a stick, and it will determine your body's pH levels, so you can adjust as necessary.

DEEP CORE STRESS HYGIENE

To begin building new, nonreactive habits around stress, try this simple stress-combating exercise the next time you catch yourself in a moment of clutching.

Gently ground down through your feet and twist your body side to side, allowing your arms to swing and head to turn, to help wring out your organs and deep belly and free up any stuck and stagnant energy in the belly. Inhale through your nose as you twist to one side, then exhale through your mouth as you twist to the other. Repeat this 10 times alternating sides.

EAT FOR BALANCE

Your dietary choices can have a major impact on your pH levels. Ideally, you want to maximize alkaline foods and reduce your consumption of highly acidic choices. Following is a quick guide to help you achieve your perfect pH balance.

Highly Alkaline Foods

- Cucumber
- Greens
- Parsley
- Spinach
- Sprouted beans

Moderately Alkaline Foods

- Arugula
- Avocado
- Garlic
- Ginger
- Grains, such as quinoa
- Lemons
- Lime

Moderately Acidic Foods

- Apples
- Blackberries
- Blueberries
- Fish

- Grapes
- Mangos
- Pineapple
- Strawberries

- Wild rice
- Wholemeal pasta

Highly Acidic Foods

- Alcohol
- Artificial sweeteners
- Cheese
- Chicken
- Coffee

- Eggs
- Meat
- Mushrooms
- Sugar
- Tea

Movement Medicine for the Deep Core

Through movement targeting the deep core, we can massage our organs and create more space to move them back to their proper alignment. We can create a sense of greater connection with our deep core in order to cultivate awareness of our hunger levels and our gut instincts.

At first, some of these moves might feel a little intense, but the results are worth it. When incorporated into your routine on a regular basis, you will enjoy healthier digestion, alleviation of lower back pain, improved posture, and a flatter, more connected belly. When you breathe into, roll, or massage your belly, it sends a signal to your nervous system to relax. It even helps reduce anxiety, decrease inflammation, stimulate the vagus nerve, and improve breathing. Belly rolling can also create an abdominal massage that mobilizes the deeper layers of the fascia, also known as connective tissues, in the core and even around the organs, freeing up and flushing the deep core and waist.

Belly Breath with Control and Surrender

This practice will assist with lower belly connection and sacral mobility.

To begin, lie face-down, resting on your forearms with a squishy ball placed under the center of your pubic bone. Take a few full breaths here to allow your body to relax and melt over the ball. This melting will release your sacrum, lower back, and organs.

Once you have fully relaxed your belly, take a full inhale to expand and release any tension or blocked energy in your deep core. Next, exhale as you curl your tail under and contract your

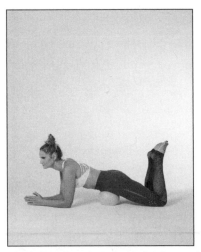 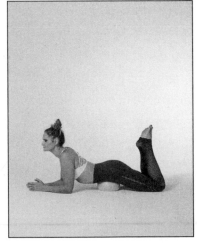

Belly Breath with Control and Surrender

lower abs, then inhale as you extend your tailbone back and stretch the front of your core. Repeat this movement 8 times.

Mid-Belly Melt with Twist

Belly rolling is the equivalent of a healing lymphatic massage. It mobilizes the fascia and organs, letting them move in a more fluid, relaxed, and graceful way.

Lie face-down, resting on your forearms with the squishy ball placed under your belly button. Keep the ball in place as you take 3 deep, full breaths. On each exhale, feel your tissues melt into the ball.

Continue to keep the ball stable and take an inhale as you twist your upper body to the left. Then exhale as you twist your upper body to the right, massaging your mid-belly and aligning your psoas. Repeat this full movement 3 times.

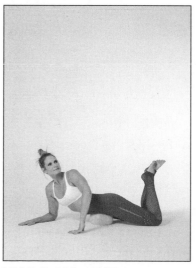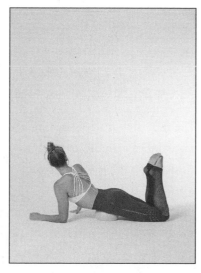

Mid-Belly Melt with Twist

De-Bloat Massage

Lie face-down and place the ball under your pubic bone. Put the palms of your hands down on the floor with your elbows bent in by your sides. Inhale as you roll up the entire front of your core to your diaphragm. Next, exhale as you roll back down to your starting position. Repeat this movement 8 times.

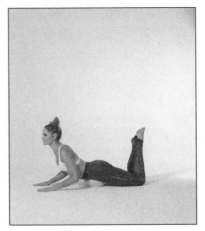 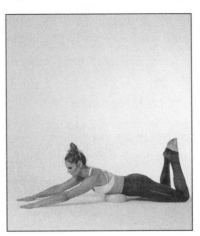

De-Bloat Massage

Psoas Massage

Lie face-down with the ball under your right psoas and then bend your left knee and extend it out to the side. Place your forearms down with elbows facing outward. Take a few deep breaths as you allow your body to soften over the ball. Next, inhale to fill up your lungs and then exhale as you roll the ball up the front of your hip and core. Then inhale as you roll the ball down your tissues, clearing out blocked energy in the deep core. Repeat 8 times each side.

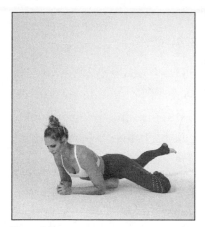

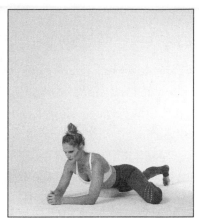

Psoas Massage

Sacral Roll

Sit with your tailbone on the squishy ball, arms reaching behind you and palms on the floor. Take a big breath in, filling up your lungs and expanding your pelvic floor, and then exhale as you curl your tail under as the ball rolls up your sacrum and lower back. Exhale as you roll the ball back down. Repeat this full series of movements 10 times.

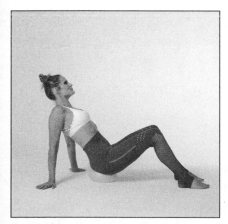

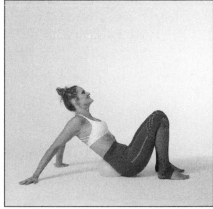

Sacral Roll

Deep Core Detoxification Breathwork

Come down to a comfortable seated position on a squishy ball or pillow. Close your eyes and feel yourself ground down into the earth. Take a deep, slow, steady breath, inhaling for a count of 8, filling up your belly, lungs, and middle back. Even when you think you can't inhale anymore, try to sip a bit more air in. Breathe all the way down into your pelvic floor and stomach, expand the lungs fully, and bring the breath all the way up into your head. This allows oxygen to reach the deepest depths of your lungs to inflate the alveoli and free up toxins and pollutants that may have accumulated in your system. When you've sipped in all the air you can, hold your breath for a count of 5, and then exhale for a count of 10. Keep flushing out the carbon dioxide from the deepest depths of your lungs and wringing out your organs. You will feel your chest and belly flatten and pull in and up.

Repeat this breathing technique 10 times. Doing this daily will help flush your body of toxins, boost metabolism, increase your lung capacity, improve digestion, boost energy, and help relieve excess stress. You'll feel the benefits immediately.

Heal and Balance Your Deep Core

Take a Moment

As we all know by now, meditation is helpful for innumerable reasons. For the purpose of this book, though, meditating is most helpful for the deep core because it allows us to get out of fight-or-flight mode. Through slowing the breath and focusing the attention, meditation can help us to bring ourselves into the present moment, where we can feel and enjoy more. When we are in the present moment, we can take better stock of our emotions and instincts without judgment.

Meditation doesn't have to mean sitting on a cushion in lotus position. It can be anything that allows you to get in a clear, present state. For some people, this might be walking or running. For others, it might be swimming. And for others, it might actually be the more traditional practice of sitting and tuning in. The goal here is to be present. How you get there is less important.

A meditative state is very healing. It gets you out of adrenal fatigue and into rest-and-digest mode. It can even help you lose weight by reducing anxiety (and, thus, cortisol) and helping you feel self-possessed and confident. It draws you inward and connects you to your truest self.

Get in Touch with Your Circadian Rhythm

In the animal world, creatures who are not nocturnal sleep when it's dark and wake up when it gets light. They do this naturally because they are in touch with Earth's electromagnetic energy, or the energy of the force created by our planet spinning.

Whether on a temporary basis (such as when we travel to a different time zone) or on a regular basis (because of work, children, social life, etc.), so many of us are out of touch with nature's rhythm. We are no different than animals, though. In fact, we *are* animals. We, too, are designed to synch up with the patterns of nature. But various factors have gotten us out of our natural cycle, ranging from too much screen time and scrolling, over-reactive stress, and overload.

We need sleep for healthy and hydrated tissues, robust digestion, immunity, metabolism, secretion of melatonin, and better stress management. Those pre-midnight hours are particularly precious when it comes to getting all of these systems up and running in their most robust state. We are *meant* to be seizing that time. Did you know that every hour you sleep before midnight is the equivalent of two hours' sleep rather than one? Make a point of turning off your screens and winding down once the sun has set. You may not go to bed at eight, but you also shouldn't be going to bed after midnight.

To get yourself into a more natural sleep rhythm, try these tips.

1. Spend some of the light hours out in nature and breathe in fresh air on a regular basis. This will help you get in tune with Earth's electromagnetic energy.
2. Magnesium before bed can lead to a sounder, more restful sleep—I like Natural Calm, which you can find on Amazon. According to the National Center for Biotechnology Information, up to 80 percent of us are magnesium deficient.
3. Pull out your journal before bed and empty all of the thoughts, stresses, and to-dos rattling around your head. This allows you to get the "buzz" out so that you can drift off to sleep with a clear mind.
4. Try sleeping on your side with your knees bent slightly upward to your chest. This allows your spine to decompress and promotes cerebrospinal circulation, which gives your

brain time to rest and heal. If you experience back pain, try putting a pillow between your legs to alleviate pressure in your hips and lower back.

5. Finally, establish a pattern, which will eventually turn into a habit. Go to sleep and get up at the same time every day. Before long, you may find that you don't even need an alarm clock anymore. Your body will fall into a natural, aligned rhythm.

Get in the Flow

Since the sacral chakra is a water element, we heal and balance our deep core by aligning with the fluid nature of water. This might mean literally spending time in or around water—sitting or swimming in a body of water or taking a bath.

But, of course, water isn't the only way to experience fluidity. We can find a fluid or flow state when we let ourselves go in activities like art, dance, or poetry. Whenever we connect through our emotions and allow our creativity to flow up through the pelvic floor, we are experiencing a flow within ourselves. As an added benefit, dance, specifically, allows us to open up our hips and get energy into and moving through the deep core. Whenever we move this part of the body, we connect with it, which is precisely what we want to accomplish as we build awareness of our deep core.

Not all cultures have tight pelvic floors like Americans tend to. One giveaway is how people in other cultures move. For instance, if you look at the average Brazilian, they love to swing their hips from side to side, whether they are walking or dancing. With this, they are opening up, expanding, and releasing their pelvic floor. It's no mistake that we also tend to think of Brazilians as sensual and sexy—they come from a culture that is deeply attentive and connected to the pelvic floor.

Take a few minutes out of your day to crank up some music and let loose. Let your hips sway from side to side and feel the rhythm. When you finish, notice how you feel, not only physically, but also emotionally and mentally. My guess is that, even after a few minutes, you'll feel happier and less stressed.

Get Comfortable with Self-Pleasure

This one may be a bit awkward to discuss or even think about due to society's somewhat Puritanical views on open discourse about masturbation. But our sex organs are just like any other area of the body. Once you can release the mental stigma around them, you can enjoy your incredible body in ways you never have before. The more you enjoy your body, the more you will appreciate it, and the better you will treat it. You will start to view your body as the sacred vessel it is.

Trust me on this one: pleasuring yourself will help you connect with yourself, your power, and your sensuality. It will allow you to reach new depths of trust, pleasure, and surrender within yourself. I highly recommend that you start slow if this concept makes you feel uncomfortable. Create a sacred, private, safe space for your self-pleasure ritual and listen to your body. Over time, you'll slowly notice your sensuality unfolding like a lotus, and pleasure will come to you much more easily in all areas of your life.

TAKE A BEAUTIFYING MILK AND HONEY BATH

The more beautiful we feel, the more sensual we become. You've probably heard of Cleopatra and her legendary beauty. Cleopatra made a regular habit of bathing in milk, honey, and roses to nourish and heal her skin.

The lactic acid in milk is an alpha hydroxy acid, which helps exfoliate and cleanse the skin to remove dead skin cells. This exfoliation paves a quick road to the sort of radiant, glowing skin every woman wants. The honey highlights this effect by softening, moisturizing, and generally beautifying the skin. Combined, these soothing ingredients will heal your skin and relax your mind.

To prepare:

1 to 2 cups full-fat or powdered milk (full-fat moisturizes the skin)

½ cup raw honey mixed with 1 cup of boiled water to liquefy the honey

Draw your bath and pour the milk and honey under the running warm water. Mix it around in the tub, and then luxuriate in this ancient, skin-healing remedy.

Mantra and Visualization for the Deep Core

*"I am a sensual and powerful being who expresses my
creative power by leading a fulfilling, joyful, pleasurable, and
passionate life."*

Find a comfortable position in which your pelvic floor can feel supported, sitting with legs crossed on a cushion, roller, or squishy ball. Come to a nice, tall, easy spine. Bring your energy and awareness into your belly and sacral area, into your gut, and into your psoas. Visualize how your psoas looks like two pillars of strength in front of your spine, holding your spine up by separating your ribs from your hips.

In front of the psoas are your beautiful organs that help nourish, heal, and cleanse your body. Allow those organs to drop down to the base of your core so they are sitting deeply in the earth. Work on letting your pelvic floor relax downward, releasing any clutching and tightness. By doing this, your organs can drop down into the hammock of your pelvic floor. Now, feel your energy moving upward effortlessly with the strength of the psoas.

Allow space between the organs so your digestive process can occur with more ease. Imagine your metabolism churning along, your adrenals calming down, and all of your systems being regulated from the inside out.

Now see your abdominal muscles, wrapping circularly around your core like a tree trunk. Imagine all of these layers from the inside out.

Allow the energy around your core to soften. Feel yourself connect more deeply to your gut instincts and inner knowing. Imagine your vagus nerve acting as a direct line from your belly to your brain. Connect to the energy of surrender in your belly area so that you can get the signals you desire to your brain and vice versa. The more you can connect to the inner sensations of what your body is telling you—what you feel when you meet someone, when you walk into the room, go for a job interview, or drive your car— the greater your sensuality superpower is. This is the superpower of making better decisions and living with more pleasure.

When you make better decisions, you can experience more joy and feel safer. You can be vulnerable. When you open up this energy of enjoyment and pleasure in a relaxed way, you can enjoy the beauty of life. You can have more fun, be more at peace, and feel more connected.

Imagine a switch and flip it on. Find presence and feel the brain-body connection of messages so that you can hear when you are full and when you truly are hungry. Giving your body more space in this area allows everything to come into alignment.

It also allows you to connect to your deeper muscles, which will give you more support from the inside out. By releasing the tension in this area and allowing the psoas and the guts to support your spine, core, and your whole body in gravity, the lower pressure is released from your back. Your hips relax and you come into a more aligned, uplifted posture.

Bring your awareness down to the pelvic floor again. Feel it release. This is your foundation for creating space, building strength, and creating a deeper connection to your gut and belly, and to sensuality.

Feel the connection between these two centers. Feel how they support one another, almost like domes, one on top of the other.

Inhale deeply, then exhale fully. Roll your shoulders up to your ears and back down. Roll your hands and your feet, straighten your legs out, and release the bend of your knees. Feel your body and release your body.

Open your eyes and notice the freedom in your body and connection to your true self.

Activate Your Sensuality Superpower Through the Deep Core

We don't often think of sensuality and intuition as being interconnected, but they are. This intersection occurs in our deep core.

Sensuality is our birthright. It has the potential to make life more enjoyable when we nurture it properly. It provides us with the ability to connect to, awaken, and embody pleasure through sight, taste, smell, touch, and sound.

When we get in touch with our deep core, we also become more attuned to our sensuality. The type of sensuality I'm referencing here involves much more than just sex. While that type of sensuality can be fun to experience, it's not a superpower. The type of deep, rich sensuality we have access to through our deep core encompasses how we connect, feel about, and interact with the people, things, and events in our lives. In this context, sensuality is very connected to intuition, connection, and charisma. It can be what we often refer to as intuition, or gut instinct—which makes sense, since our gut is connected to our deep core. I'm talking about the physical signals we've all experienced as we interact with the world. The gut acts as intuition's sensory system. I'm sure you've experienced these sensations plenty of times in your own life—the butterflies that flutter in your stomach when you're excited about someone or something, or the niggling discomfort you feel in your belly when something is a bit "off." These physical cues occur because we carry a lot of emotion in our belly. At the end of the day, intuition is emotion. There are other ways of connecting with intuition, but the gut is where it speaks the most loudly and clearly.

ALTERNATIVE THERAPIES FOR THE DEEP CORE

Aromatherapy: Ylang Ylang

Sourced from a tropical tree in Indonesia, Malaysia, and the Philippines, ylang ylang has the sort of sultry, floral aroma you would expect from these regions. It smells deliciously romantic, but that's only the beginning of what ylang ylang has to offer. The scent is thought to be able to assist in everything from calming nerves to lifting the mood to managing emotional well-being, and even elevating the libido.

Ylang ylang will have the greatest effect on your deep core when you rub a few drops from your belly button down to the top of your pubic bone. You can also inhale it from the bottle or diffuse it to help you remain in the current moment.

Crystals

I like all of these crystals for the deep core because, while they each offer specific benefits, they all commonly reconnect you with your gut instincts, renew your ability to feel and sense, and heal your organs.

- **Carnelian**—harmonizes mental focus and creativity and helps you put plans into action with confidence
- **Orange calcite**—breaks old patterns, overcomes shyness, and sparks creative fire
- **Pink tourmaline**—strengthens the sense of smell and enhances the perception and awareness of pheromones

To heal your deep core, select the crystal that resonates with you most and place it between your belly button and pubic bone. As it rests there, meditate, relax, or visualize the outcome you hope to receive. For a more consistent infusion of healing vibes, you can also carry your selected crystal with you in your purse or pocket, wear it as jewelry, or place it in your home or car.

I particularly like to place crystals in my bedroom so that I can receive their healing benefits while I sleep. This is a particularly potent way to use crystals, because when we sleep our subconscious mind kicks into gear and deep healing occurs. Try placing the crystal either under your pillow or on the side of your bed. Observe how your dreams are affected and notice if you feel more rested the next morning.

Tea

This healing combination of lemon, fennel, and ginger is the perfect tea to de-bloat your belly, improve digestion, and cleanse the body of toxins. It may even help with weight loss. The result is a flatter, happier belly.

To prepare:

2 cups water
½ teaspoon crushed fennel seeds
1 fresh ginger root, washed, peeled, and cut into small pieces
Juice of 1 lemon

Add the water, fennel seeds, and ginger root into a small saucepan and bring to a boil for 10 minutes. Pour the hot water through a strainer and add the lemon juice. This tea is best enjoyed after a meal.

Nourish Your Deep Core

Herbs for the Deep Core

TURMERIC

Turmeric is a brilliant anti-inflammatory, anti-bacterial, and antioxidant-packed herb that is said to help boost immunity and stimulate proper digestion. Be sure to mix it with a bit of black pepper to increase bioavailability and reap its full benefits.

DIGESTIVE ENZYMES

Digestive enzymes help your body absorb more of the good nutrients from your food and eliminate elements that are not so good for you. Our bodies naturally make enzymes to improve digestion and break down foods. However, as we age—and, particularly if we are under large amounts of stress—our enzyme levels can decrease, which leads to digestive imbalances.

Research shows that broad-spectrum enzymes can help break

down lactose, proteins, carbohydrates, fibers, and fats to help improve digestion and keep your belly happy. But even if you're not experiencing these issues, digestive enzymes are beneficial for everyone. Just pop one of these before you eat and you will notice the difference. I love Hum Nutrition Flatter Me Digestive Enzymes, which can be found at www.humnutrition.com.

Minerals for the Deep Core: Magnesium

Soil in the United States has been depleted from over-farming. Specifically, our soil lacks magnesium, which can help reduce stress and calm the nervous system.

My favorite brand is Natural Calm, a nonpowdered, flavored form of magnesium. I like to add it to 16 ounces of warm water and drink it before bed. Make sure that whatever brand you take is bioavailable for optimal absorption.

FOODS THAT HEAL THE DEEP CORE

- **Fermented foods**—kimchi and yogurt
- **Good fats**—foods such as avocados and extra-virgin olive oil help raise your vibration, radiancy, and vitality levels
- **Orange-colored foods**—apricots, carrots, mangos, papaya, pumpkin

---

Sensuality Tonic

MAKES 16 OUNCES

If the bright color of this tonic isn't enough to get you going, the energizing raw maca powder definitely will. Maca can help reduce stress, boost nourishment, increase stamina, combat fatigue, and seems to improve sexual function for both men and women. Carrots are a well-known libido enhancer that increase sex hormones, promote fertility, and are loaded with vitamin A. The cayenne increases good sensations and will get your blood flowing in all of the right places.

16 carrots
1 tablespoon maca powder
Dash of cayenne pepper
Pinch of Himalayan salt

Juice the carrots. Transfer the fresh juice into a blender, add the maca and cayenne, and blend for about 30 seconds. Pour the juice into a glass and top with the Himalayan salt.

Stimulating Sparkling Kefir Elixir

MAKES 32 OUNCES

According to ancient Chinese medicine, ginger has the ability to "build fire" in the belly for better digestion and increased sensuality. It is also commonly used in spells to enhance magical powers and attract love and success. This blend will seduce with its probiotic powers and captivating, refreshing zing. This will take 24 hours to ferment, so be sure to plan ahead!

3 cups raw coconut water (I like Harmless Harvest)
½ cup freshly squeezed orange juice
1 packet kefir starter (I like Body Ecology)
1 tablespoon ginger root, peeled and freshly grated

Add the coconut water and orange juice to a small saucepan on low heat. Heat to lukewarm and remove from heat. Combine this mixture with the kefir starter in a quart-size mason jar. Add the ginger and stir to mix well.

Place the lid on the mason jar and allow the blend to ferment at room temperature for 24 hours (or up to 48 if you prefer a tangier blend).

This elixir can be stored in the refrigerator (40 to 50 degrees F) for up to 2 to 3 weeks, or in the freezer (0 to 25 degrees F) for 1 to 2 months.

Soothing Belly Broth

MAKES 8 TO 10 BOWLS

This cup of nourishment for the soul is a beautiful, soothing, gut-healing blend filled with minerals that will nourish all of your cells and tissues. Studies are showing that just one cup of broth a day, whether on its own or as a base, has a significant impact on belly health, healthy skin, inflammation, and immunity.

    32 ounces organic bone broth
    4 celery stalks, chopped
    10 ounces spinach
    5 basil leaves
    3 cloves garlic, crushed
    1 inch ginger, peeled and roughly chopped
    avocado, sliced (optional to garnish)

Pour the bone broth into a large pot. Add in the celery, spinach, basil, garlic, and ginger. Simmer over medium heat for 30 minutes, or until the vegetables are soft. Pour the soup into a blender and blend until you have achieved a smooth consistency.

Garnish with avocado to serve.

5

The Upper Core Power Center: The Confidence Superpower

SIGNS YOUR UPPER CORE NEEDS SOME LOVE

Physical

* Consistently low levels of energy
* A sluggish metabolism
* You need coffee, sugar, or stimulants to get going

* Inability to take a full, deep breath, or always feeling out of breath
* Tension or tightness in your middle back, around the bottom of the shoulder blades

Emotional

* Feeling of misalignment or a lack of purpose in life
* Trying to control or manipulate others

* Lack of confidence
* Fear of taking risks in life or pushing beyond comfort zone

The Imbalanced Upper Core

Zach is a professional hockey player who was looking for a competitive edge. He wanted to differentiate his training regime from that of his teammates and opponents, so he came to me. As a professional hockey player, Zach was in great shape, but his body had suffered some wear and tear from constant exertion and repetitive movement. His entire trunk and rib cage were rotated, with one shoulder forward. As a result, he lacked the ability to take a full breath, often felt exhausted, and couldn't recover quickly. He was young, but pretty banged up.

The compressed rib cage, inability to take a deep breath, and exhaustion prompted me to zero in on Zach's upper core. We went into his diaphragm and found a lot of tension there, which he was entirely unaware of (as are 99.9 percent of the population). This tension was impeding Zach's lung capacity, which is crucial in competitive sports.

Zach and I started focusing on the compressed space and worked to release stress in his diaphragm through a combination of breathwork and movement medicine. Very quickly, Zach felt more energized due to the increased oxygen flow. Deeper breaths also kicked up his ability to recover, and even boosted his metabolism. We were able to get rid of the hunch behind Zach's diaphragm, which—in addition to his quicker metabolism— changed his shape. He became taller and more narrow. His movements grew more fluid and efficient. He used to joke with me that he was going to send me his tailor's bills for all of the suits he had to get taken in.

As a result of this work on his upper core, Zach felt more

confident in his body, game, career, and in general. He felt like he had found that edge he was looking for.

Get to Know Your Upper Core

The upper core is located in the upper trunk of our torso, right in the center of our body. It consists of our diaphragm and lungs, which expand three-dimensionally into our middle back, below the shoulder blades. Our adrenal glands are also found here.

When your upper core is imbalanced, you will likely notice lower levels of energy, slower metabolism and digestion, and difficulty sleeping. Anxiety, nausea, a quickened heartbeat, feelings of restlessness and overwhelm, and the inability to take a deep breath are also indicative of issues in the upper core.

In the human body, a complex collection of nerves in one specific location is known as a "plexus," which means network. The upper core includes a plexus—located in that soft area right below your breastbone. Western medicine refers to this as the celiac (or abdominal) plexus. It is a juncture point of nerves in the abdomen, near the stomach. The plexus found in the upper core is one of the main plexuses in the human body. This network means that anything that affects the upper core can cause significant problems throughout our entire system. If you've ever had the wind knocked out of you, that's an effect of a blow to the upper core. The blow irritates a nerve in the nearby diaphragm, causing it to spasm. Since the diaphragm is essential to breathing, you can't take a full breath until the effect wears off.

Mystics have claimed the upper core is the center of our emotions. While medical science doesn't explain it in the same terms, it has found the upper core to be a physically vulnerable point in the body where interconnecting nerves can be irritated, which causes pain. Nerves included in the upper core include those that govern the autonomic nervous system, that part of the nervous system that we don't voluntarily control. The autonomic nervous system regulates organ function, constriction and dilation of blood vessels, and pupil size.

In this chapter, we will focus a lot on the quality of breath. Breathing deeply and fully impacts our physical health in profound ways, and it's also one of the most accessible tools at our disposal to regulate stress. In order to tap into all the benefits that great breathing has to offer, we will need a solid understanding of the diaphragm. The diaphragm is a dome-shaped muscle located at the bottom of the rib cage. It separates our chest from our abdominal capacity, and dwells in the thoracic part of our body (the circumference of the upper-back area), which also contains the heart and lungs. Closely connected to the digestive system, the main function of the diaphragm is to help transform matter into energy to fuel your body. It governs metabolism and is commonly associated with the pancreas.

When our diaphragm contracts, it expands the length and diameter of the chest cavity, which allows the lungs to expand. When the diaphragm expands, it presses down on the pelvic floor and contracts the length and diameter of the chest cavity, which allows the lungs to compress—and thus creates the mechanics of our inhalations and exhalations. Through this functionality, our diaphragm is responsible for the oxygen we take in and the carbon monoxide we breathe out. It goes without saying: this is an essential function of life.

Our lungs have the capacity to take in approximately two

gallons of oxygen at a time; however, most of us utilize only 20 to 30 percent of that capacity. Stop and think about that for a minute: the vast majority of us are taking in just a small percentage of life force that is available to us.

Obviously, this brings with it a whole host of problems. For the purposes of our physicality, though, deep breaths are important for deep core strength and to release tension or stress. The process of breathing helps us connect to the deep layers of our core. It is these layers that draw the belly musculature in and up. If you can't quite visualize this, these are the same muscles we feel when we laugh or cough really hard. They are also the muscles that support our spine and diaphragm. They help keep us uplifted and inspired, because the way we hold ourselves has a direct impact on our mood and state of mind.

Perhaps you've noticed a pattern throughout your body by now: whenever something is tight, it weakens and impedes efficient functioning. The same is true of the diaphragm. Our stomach is located directly under the diaphragm and lungs, so anything happening in our diaphragm impacts our stomach and organs. When our diaphragm is tight, it compresses our organs, which prevents them from functioning optimally, and prevents our blood from flowing freely.

The Upper Core and Holistic Health

Professional and competitive athletes spend a lot of time doing diaphragm work, because it allows them to perform at higher levels and enhances their endurance. They are training themselves to breathe more fully and effectively and recover more efficiently. The more fresh oxygen they bring in, the better they can nourish their cells. In the absence of deep breath, our metabolism is sluggish, our energy levels are lower, and our ability to deal with stress decreases drastically.

Your breath is also a great tool for weight loss. To this day, many health professionals are still mystified about how we actually lose weight. There is a direct correlation between how we exhale and weight loss, because our exhalation boosts metabolism. Fat is converted to carbon dioxide and water, so almost everything we eat comes back out via the lungs. If you lose 10 pounds of fat, 8.4 pounds comes out through your lungs, and 1.6 pounds comes out as water.

This explains why so many people are frustrated about their inability to lose weight. No matter how much you diet or work out, if your lungs, ribs, intercostals, and diaphragm are glued down by tight, rigid fascia, you're not going to be able to let out the deep, expansive breaths weight loss requires. All of the breath exercises included in the Movement Medicine section of this book will result in this type of deep, expansive breath. Stay tuned for the additional benefit of weight loss as you put these breathing techniques into practice.

The Solar Plexus Chakra

The solar plexus chakra, which is appropriately associated with the color yellow, is representative of the fire in our belly. It is located around the pancreas, the part of the body that controls our metabolism.

The main function of the solar plexus is to power our life with forward motion. It helps us to realize our personal desires and clarifies our intentions. Appropriately, this chakra both tasks and assists us with discovering our confidence, which will, in turn, provide us with the momentum we need to walk down our optimal life path, no matter how daunting it may seem at times. The solar plexus propels us toward our goals.

When we experience the sort of confidence the solar plexus helps us cultivate, we can be assertive without being overbearing. We can accept our failures with the understanding that they, too, are part of our process and draw us closer to our ultimate aims.

In this chakra, we learn that confidence is the furthest thing from selfishness. It is only through cultivating confidence and self-direction that we can share our greatest gifts and offerings with the world in their fullest form. This benefits not only you, but everyone whose life you touch.

The Upper Core and the Pelvic Floor

You can think of your body as a series of three boxes stacked one on top of the other: the pelvic floor, the diaphragm, and the jaw. Just like an entire stack of boxes is thrown off-kilter if they aren't properly aligned, such is the case with your body. If your pelvic floor, diaphragm, or jaw is locked up or pulled down through the weight of compression, the others will be, too. Whatever we experience in one "box" will be mirrored in the structure and stability of the other boxes. If your pelvic floor is tight and congested, you can be sure your diaphragm will be, too.

Located toward the middle of the body, the diaphragm impacts not only what is below it, but also what is above it. If your diaphragm isn't strong and resilient, you won't be able to relax your shoulders down your back efficiently and effortlessly. Instead, you will end up hunched over. Think of your diaphragm as a deep core muscle and visualize it as a hydraulic system, which moves material through the application of pressure. With the "pressure" of breath, your diaphragm pumps oxygen in and CO_2 out of your body. As the diaphragm contracts, air volume increases, pressing down into your pelvic floor and expanding into the lungs. If your pelvic floor is tight, the diaphragm can't push down as much air, nor can you let as much out. You will never be able to release and expand your diaphragm without also doing the same in the pelvic floor, and vice versa. Not only is this unhealthy—not to mention uncomfortable—from a physical standpoint, but it also runs in direct opposition to your ability to connect with your superpower of confidence.

The Upper Core and Stress

When we're stressed, it shows in our breath. Or, rather, it shows through our *lack* of breath.

Our breath becomes short and stuck when we are in a reactive state of fear, worry, or tension. But the key is that the breath is the one big thing we can actually control through awareness and with the tools in this book. We can actually train new patterns to help our bodies and minds thrive in these situations and no longer be victims.

The manner in which we breathe impacts our nervous system. Remember our old friend, the vagus nerve? Our diaphragm sends a message to the vagus nerve telling it to calm down (or not). This message is then zipped up to our brain, which triggers a reaction throughout our entire nervous system.

These messages are sent through our breath. How empowering is that? It means we have the ability to alter our levels of stress by choosing to breathe in a different way. When we change our breath, we change our entire state. When we take deep, full breaths, both our heart rate and blood pressure lower.

Stop for a moment and notice how you are breathing right now. Your breath holds a lot of clues about who you are and how you interact with the world. I have noticed this pervasive pattern in my clients: when a person overly emphasizes their exhales, they are likely depressed, defeated, and hunched over; when they overly emphasize their inhales, they are most likely a yes-person who tries too hard. These patterns show up due to feeling the weight of the world on our shoulders, or the overly erect posture of trying to control too many things and never really enjoying presence or the fruits of our labor. Does this resonate with you? Now, think about shifting your breath, lengthening out your inhales and exhales, and executing each of them fully. Breathe all the way in as you inhale, and gently allow the air to release all the way out as you exhale. Continue this pattern of breath for one minute. Notice if you can feel a shift in your stress levels. In the truest sense, your breath can transform your life.

Through our breath, we want to find that optimal middle ground of expansion and release. Your breath will bring you into the moment. It will remind you about the things you want to bring into your world and the things you want to let go. It will allow you to maximize your enjoyment of life. And it will most certainly ensure you do not become a victim of stress. The way we breathe is the way we live. Breathe deep.

UPPER CORE STRESS HYGIENE

To begin building new, nonreactive habits around stress, try this simple stress-combating exercise the next time you catch yourself in a moment of breath holding and clutching.

Come to a seated position and curl your fingertips underneath the sides of your rib cage and take a deep breath, and then exhale as you gently press your fingers a bit deeper to release congestion in the upper core.

Movement Medicine for the Upper Core

Diaphragm Massage

Place the ball on the mat, under your rib cage at the top of your core while you face down with your forearms under your forehead and legs reaching long. Take a few deep breaths to open and expand your upper core. Place your right hand on the floor with your thumb lined up with the ball. Inhale as you lean your upper body to the right, allowing the squishy ball to roll toward your breast bone. Exhale and press into your right palm, rolling the ball back over the right side of your rib cage and leaning your body to the left. Repeat this series of movements 8 times on each side.

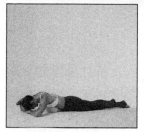
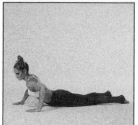
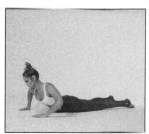

Diaphragm Massage

Upper Middle Back Extension

Lie down on your mat face-up and place the ball behind your middle back. Bend your knees and place your feet on the floor, hips-width distance apart. Bring your hands behind your head to support your neck. Inhale as you arch back, opening up your diaphragm and lungs. Exhale as you rock your upper body to the right. Inhale as you come to center and then exhale as you rock to the left, allowing the ball to softly massage your upper back, opening up your diaphragm and lungs. Repeat this series of movements 8 times.

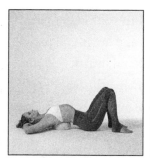
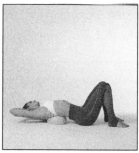
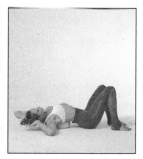

Upper Middle Back Extension

Upper Back Ball Roll

Lie down on the mat with your knees bent, feet on the floor, and place the ball under your middle back. Bring your hands behind your head with your elbows wide. Inhale as you lift your hips up and press into your feet to roll the ball down your back. Exhale as you roll the ball up your back while your knees draw over your toes. Repeat this series of movements 8 times.

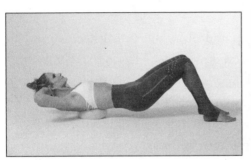
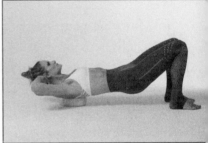

Upper Back Ball Roll

Side Rib Breathing

Come down onto the mat on your right hip with your knees beat. Place the ball under the right side of your ribs and lungs and place your right elbow on the mat. Place your left hand in front of you on the mat. Inhale as you arch your spine, allowing the ball to roll behind you. Exhale as you curl your tailbone under, rolling the side rib cage to create elasticity in the ribs and lungs. Repeat this series of movements 8 times on each side.

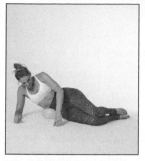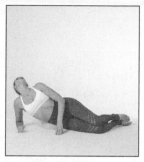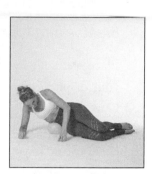

Side Rib Breathing

Extend Surrender Pose

Place the ball under your upper middle back. Extend your legs long, open your heart, and extend your arms behind you. Inhale and feel your lungs expand. Exhale as you release tension, letting the ball gently sink into your tissue. Take 10 long, deep breaths from this position.

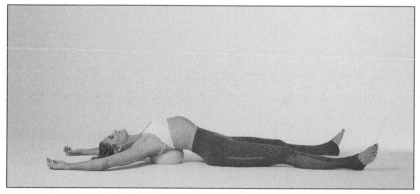

Extend Surrender Pose

Breathe into Your Upper Core

Place the squishy ball on your mat and lie face-down so that your diaphragm is on the ball and your forearms are on the mat. Gaze forward, allowing the ball to melt into your tissues. Shake your hips gently from side to side to release tension in your lower back. Inhale as you slide your elbows out to the side, allowing the squishy ball to deepen into your body. Exhale and lay your forehead down on your hands. Inhale as you expand your breath into your upper back. Exhale, allowing the ball to sink deeper into your diaphragm. Repeat this series 8 to 10 times.

Heal and Balance Your Upper Core

Take a Self-Defense Class

No matter what modality of self-defense you choose to practice, it is an ideal way to get your heart and blood pumping. It will stoke the fire in your belly. It will strengthen you not only physically, but also mentally and emotionally.

We empower ourselves with confidence through the knowledge that we are capable and safe in the world. When we know we can defend ourselves, fear falls by the wayside. Self-defense practices also teach us to own our power and to take up space in the world. It is the physical manifestation of "not playing small."

Take Up More Space

Speaking of taking up more space in the world, the practice of making room for ourselves in a physical sense is extremely transformative and an incredibly powerful confidence builder.

So many of us—particularly women—physically shrink ourselves down. It is almost impossible to act with confidence when we hold ourselves in this way. Own your space and your presence. If this doesn't come naturally to you, it might seem like an overwhelming habit to cultivate, but it is entirely possible with practice—and probably easier than you would imagine.

When you walk into a room, ground down through your pinky toe, big toe, and heel, while simultaneously lifting up through your torso and softening your shoulders down to carry yourself with a graceful and elegant posture. Feel the support of the earth beneath you, flowing up through your body and empowering you. Take a deep breath in and, as you exhale, intentionally release everything—your jaw, your belly, and your hips. Walk with relaxed confidence and the intention of connecting and making a difference. Own your energy. Claim your presence. Revel in being you, walking your path, and in being where you are in this moment.

Soak in Some Vitamin D

The upper core loves the sun because it is located in our solar plexus. Soaking up some rays will not only heal and balance your solar plexus area, but it's also a great way to absorb some Vitamin D.

Vitamin D is only available to us in two forms—from the sun

and as a supplement. The human body does not naturally produce this hormone. Vitamin D helps combat anxiety and depression, which is why people who live in gray climates often suffer from depression.

Walk outside and feel the sunshine beating on your back, do some gardening on a sunny day, or take a nice relaxing snooze in a park or your backyard. Or perhaps you're able to plan your day to make room to witness a sunset or sunrise. Allow yourself to be fully present in the moment. Absorb the yellow, orange, red, and pink hues, and allow them to stimulate your soul. Feel your mind clear as you watch the sun make its slow but steady rise or descent. As you watch the sun rise, think about the things you want to start or bring into your life. As you watch it set, think about the things you can let go that are taking up valuable space or preventing you from walking your path.

The great thing about this practice is that you can make it energizing or relaxing, depending upon how you most prefer your Vitamin D served up on any given day.

LOL

When we think of confidence, we often associate it with a self-important, serious, or even stern demeanor. In my opinion, nothing could be further from the truth. Few things are as empowering as enjoying a good, hearty laugh.

Humor reminds us that life is constantly in transition. There are few things that make you feel more helpless than trying to fight against the natural tide of life. When we act with confidence, we cease fighting the flow of life. We let go of the desire to control what "should" happen. When we come to this place, we learn to find opportunities for growth when things don't go our way, rather than feeling victimized.

A hearty laugh will help you find this place of good humor and acceptance. The more difficult or stressful life feels, the more important it is not to take things too seriously. Laughing is the best core strengthener available to us, and it also helps awaken the diaphragm, which is precisely why singers and actors use it to warm up before performing. We access freedom through humor and laughter. When we are able to stop taking the things that "happen" to us so seriously, we find confidence in its truest, most graceful form.

Pump Yourself Up

Confidence isn't theoretical. It is a real thing we can discover in the present moment. What better way is there to bring yourself into the moment than by turning on some tunes, letting go, and rocking out?

Crank up some Beyoncé or whatever up-tempo music makes you feel powerful, alive, and invigorated. Belt out a tune that reminds you of a happy time in your life and allow that old feeling to flow through you. Have fun with it! Sing in the car at the top of your lungs (bonus points for rolling down the window). Dance. Tap into that energy that makes you feel strong and confident. Singing uses your diaphragm, which activates your core, and also increases the happy-making hormone serotonin and releases stressful cortisol.

TAKE A POWER-UP BATH

Legend has it that the Greek goddess Aphrodite was born in the sea and emerged from it with rosemary draped around her. Lore tells us this rosemary warded off evil spirits and dispelled negative magic.

This bath will help relieve stress, reduce sugar cravings by calming your nervous system, and encourage the body to shed excess weight. The blend also clears toxic energy, encourages mental clarity, promotes self-identity, improves self-confidence, and renews enthusiasm. All of this contributes to a healthier ego.

¼ cup dried rosemary
10 drops rosemary essential oil
2 cups Epsom salt
½ cup baking soda

To make this bath, steep the rosemary into a cup of boiling water for 5 minutes. While the rosemary is steeping, in a small bowl, mix the rosemary essential oil into the Epsom salt and baking soda. Pour the contents into your bath. When the rosemary has steeped, pour it through a strainer over the bath.

Mantra and Visualization for the Upper Core

---

*"I am positively empowered and successful in all my ventures.
I am of value."*

Find a nice, comfortable, and supported position sitting on your roller, squishy ball, or half-dome. Relax as you feel your upright spine effortlessly and gracefully holding you up tall toward the sun. Feel your sitz bones ground down, connecting you to the earth.

Bring your awareness to your ribs and diaphragm. Visualize your ribs wrapping all the way around your middle back. Visualize your diaphragm as a dome-shaped muscle that separates your chest cavity from the abdominal cavity. This beautiful umbrella-shaped muscle is responsible for how much oxygen goes into your lungs and how much CO_2 comes out.

The diaphragm is important for handling digestion and how we respond to stress. Most people in America have a tight, stiff diaphragm that doesn't have the ability to expand and contract the way that it was designed to. With that in mind, take a nice, easy breath, fill up your lungs, and then exhale. Get to know this three-dimensional muscle as you breathe out what is not serving you.

Energetically, this area has a lot to do with your personal power and how you bring that into the world. Notice if you feel yourself hunching, either physically or energetically. When we are hunched in either of these ways, it blocks our personal power.

This power is not about force. It's not about controlling others. This power is about being you—being authentic and on your own powerful path, connecting with your gifts, and making a difference in your world and in the lives of others. It is about feeling good about these gifts and this power.

Acknowledge how connecting to this part of your body can help you live a happier, more powerful, and more balanced life.

As you continue to breathe, remember that how you breathe is how you live. If you want to live a deep life in which you have the fluidity to go with the flow, this area is so important. It is here that you create the space and elasticity for it. It's here that you create expansion and compression.

For a moment, bring your awareness to the pelvic floor. See if you can relax it any amount. Shift your awareness up to your deep core. Where and how can you relax your belly? Now come back to the diaphragm. Notice if you are holding any tension right under your rib cage. Visualize softening that energy.

If you feel a disconnect to your diaphragm, know that's normal. Take your fingers and press up into your rib cage and palpate them a few times. Make a hook shape with your fingers and hook them around and up into your ribs. Take an inhale, and then exhale. As you exhale, think about surrendering and vibrate your hooked fingers against your rib cage to help loosen and relax them. Rock your fingers side to side in that same area and continue rocking your way down and then up toward the breastbone. Relax your arms. Notice if you can now feel a deeper connection to that part of your body.

Take an inhale, holding it in for a moment, and then exhale. Resume your normal pattern of breath. Notice if you feel a greater sense of expansion in your diaphragm and rib cage.

This area is such an important key to relaxing the entire body. Breath is your tool; in fact it is a superpower in and of itself. It gives you support and allows you to ride the waves of life in the most graceful, fluid way possible. It also allows you to feel grounded. It sweeps away stress and breathes life into your body, soul, heart, and mind.

Now that you are in this relaxed state, your mind and body are more open to imprinting ideas. From that place, consider this idea: *stress is a reaction*. We have a choice and the power to choose how we react. Imprint that idea into your nervous system and into your cellular vibration. Know that this choice in reaction is a superpower. You can choose to be stressed or you can choose to believe that you are on your path, doing exactly what you are meant to do. You are in the flow of life, connected to yourself and to the people and world around you. You are connected to your path.

Take a deep breath. As you exhale, notice if you feel any calmer. Feel yourself connected to your personal power and to yourself.

Activate Your Confidence Superpower Through the Upper Core

It is the ability to contract and expand in this area that allows us to effortlessly stand up tall and proud. This might sound like a small thing, but it's not. How we carry ourselves in the world directly translates to how we feel about ourselves and our place in the world. If we hold ourselves up and claim our space, we will soon begin to feel worthy and powerful. Think about it: have you ever met someone with a commanding presence who was hunched over? My guess is the answer is no.

When we stand tall, our life experience and how we interact with the world begins to change. We take action with greater confidence and assume more accountability and responsibility for where we are in life and where we're going. This stature allows for more movement and flow, and we become better attuned with ourselves and our life. With this, we gain a clearer sense of confidence and purpose. We speak from a place of conviction and strength. We command respect, not through aggression, but through the power of our presence.

It is said that how you breathe is how you live. I believe this is true. When we hold ourselves in a manner that creates more space and flow, we breathe differently. We take in more life force and exhale in a way that simultaneously grounds and centers our body and connects us with our inner knowing.

Ego is directly related to confidence and power, so our ego originates from this upper core area. I'm not talking about the type of ego we correlate with being selfish or cocky, but the ego as a source of drive and inner fire. The ego is associated with the masculine energy of doing. From this area of the body, we source the energy that powers us along our true path with a sense of focus, purpose, and confidence.

ALTERNATIVE THERAPIES FOR THE UPPER CORE

Aromatherapy

The lungs love eucalyptus and peppermint scents. Both of these uplifting yet soothing flavors are great for alleviating tightness in the lungs, as well as activating and expanding them.

Hold the eucalyptus or peppermint oil about an inch away from your nose and enjoy a nice, deep inhale. You can also add a few drops directly into your shower stream, and take a nice, steamy eucalyptus- or peppermint-scented shower. You will emerge feeling refreshed and rejuvenated. Of course, you can also diffuse these scents, either separately or together.

Crystals

The common factor among all of these crystals is that they will help you build confidence in a holistic way that has a positive impact on your mind, body, and emotional energy. This is exactly the type of support our upper core needs to thrive.

- **Amber**—cleanses, balances, and increases mental clarity and confidence
- **Citrine**—this "success stone" is used to balance, cleanse, and help with personal empowerment and confidence
- **Lemon quartz**—this "stone of optimism" is used to cleanse and activate the solar upper core
- **Yellow tourmaline**—good for detox, cleansing, and activating balance
- **Tiger's eye**—this stone offers protection, grounding, cleansing, and balance

To heal your upper core, select the crystal that resonates with you most and place it right under your chest. As it rests there, meditate, relax, or visualize the outcome you hope to receive. For a more consistent infusion of healing vibes, you can also carry your selected crystal with you in your purse or pocket, wear it as jewelry, or place it in your home or car.

Tea

Valerian root is a super-root that has been used in some cultures as a remedy for all sorts of things, including healing adrenal fatigue, restoring the nervous system, and even lowering blood pressure. It's been used for centuries to treat nervousness, heart palpitations, and even insomnia. Some early research suggests that Valerian root may produce a calming effect similar to that which anti-anxiety drugs provide. For all of these reasons, valerian root is sometimes called nature's valium.

I like to enjoy valerian root tea about an hour before heading to bed because it encourages deep, restorative beauty sleep. When taken on a nightly basis you'll be amazed at how your body begins to rebalance. (As an added benefit, your cravings for sweets will also be reduced.)

1 teaspoon dried organic valerian root

Steep the valerian root in hot water for 10 minutes. Pour the tea through a strainer and serve.

Nourish Your Upper Core

Herbs for the Upper Core

MACA

Maca is a powder made of Peruvian root. In Peru, workers and warriors used to take Maca to bolster their endurance and strength. This adaptogen is great for bringing in balance. I like to scoop some maca powder into my smoothie every morning for an extra boost of energy, stamina, and vitality to greet the day.

OREGANO

Oregano oil is a quick fix for clearing and detoxifying the lungs. I love how simple it is to incorporate oregano into pretty much any meal as a seasoning. Be aware that oregano oil packs a powerful punch, both in terms of taste and smell—but its impact is powerful as well! I've found the best way to ingest oregano oil is by adding a few drops to water and taking a shot.

ROSEMARY

Here's another easy herb to get in! Who doesn't love the taste and smell of rosemary? Not only is it delightful, but it's also a great way to detoxify the upper intestines, which produce and distribute digestive enzymes, insulin, and other hormones for radiant health. The world is your oyster here—you can get your rosemary in through tea, as a garnish, or even by dropping some tincture into water for a healing and refreshing treat.

Vitamins for the Upper Core: Vitamin D

As we've already discussed, pretty much everyone is Vitamin D deficient, since we can only obtain this hormone through the sun or supplements. In supplement form, try a sublingual yellow pellet form of Vitamin D to place under your tongue, as that is the most bioavailable form.

A much more fun way of getting your daily dose of D is spending thirty minutes in the sun without sunscreen—yes, you read that right: no sunscreen. After thirty minutes, you will absolutely want to apply sunscreen to protect your skin, but get your vitamins in first!

FOODS THAT HEAL THE UPPER CORE

- **Enzyme-filled fruits**—bananas, pineapple, and papayas
- **Spicy foods**—cinnamon, cumin, ginger, and turmeric
- **Yellow-colored foods**—chickpeas, legumes, ginger, lemons, and yellow peppers

---

Confidence-Boosting Tonic

MAKES 16 OUNCES

A nourished upper core will fill your life with more confidence, enthusiasm, joy, willpower, and motivation to act with purpose. It breeds a warm personality, playfulness, good-self-esteem, and the ability to face challenges with courage. What more motivation do you need to drink up this tonic?

The grapefruit base includes an enzyme that will help your body better utilize sugar. This boosts metabolism and aids in weight loss. It also bolsters immunity, hydrates the body, and promotes skin and brain health. In Ayurvedic medicine, grapefruit is believed to cleanse the mind and stimulate confidence, intelligence, and creativity. The addition of mint will give your metabolism an extra boost by stimulating digestive enzymes.

2 cups water
½ organic grapefruit, sliced
1 teaspoon ginger, chopped or sliced
5 to 6 mint leaves

Combine the water, grapefruit, ginger, and mint in a glass or mason jar. Allow the mixture to sit at room temperature for approximately 2 hours. To maximize the flavor, muddle the ingredients right before straining. Strain the mixture and enjoy!

Fire-Up Elixir

MAKES 8 OUNCES

I like to have this juice once a day, and sometimes twice. I find it is best absorbed on an empty stomach, so I often make it part of my morning routine to fire up my day. The watercress helps soothe swollen breathing passages and lubricates the lungs. Turnips are high in vitamin A and lemons contain vitamin C, and both are full of antioxidants and promote lung health.

1 cucumber, chopped
1 lemon, peeled and quartered
1 turnip, chopped
1 bunch watercress

Place the cucumber, lemon, turnip, and watercress in a juicer or blender and blend on high until you have achieved a liquefied texture.

If you are using a juicer, run the juice through a strainer before serving to separate the pulp.

Power-Balancing Broth

MAKES 8 TO 10 BOWLS

Stimulate your metabolism, awaken your personal power, and harness your motivation with this body-mind broth. Since the upper core is the source of our confidence, nourishing balance in this area is key to your overall sense of self-worth and happiness. This power center loves the uplifting benefits of the medicinal herb lemongrass, which is known to help regulate the adrenals and promote better circulation.

32 ounces bone broth

2 tablespoons coconut oil

2 tablespoons lemongrass, coarsely chopped

3 tablespoons cilantro leaves, chopped, plus extra for garnish

2 scallions, chopped

3 springs thyme

4 bay leaves

4 garlic cloves, chopped

Pinch of cayenne pepper, to taste

Himalayan salt, to taste

Bring the bone broth to boil and add the coconut oil, lemongrass, cilantro, scallions, thyme, bay leaves, garlic, cayenne, and salt. Reduce the heat to low, partially cover the broth, and allow it to simmer for 15 minutes. Serve hot or warmed with cilantro to garnish.

To store, allow the broth to cool to room temperature before refrigerating or freezing. Store it in an airtight glass container in the refrigerator for 5 to 7 days or in the freezer for up to 4 months.

6

The Heart and Shoulders Power Center: Unlock Your Love Superpower

SIGNS YOUR HEART AND SHOULDERS NEED SOME LOVE

Physical

* Constant tension in shoulders
* Tightness in your chest
* Shoulders scrunched up by your ears
* Tension and stiffness in the upper back
* Chronic knots between the shoulder blades
* Feeling of compression in the chest and heart

Emotional

* Feeling of the weight of the world on your shoulders
* Anxiety and depression
* Difficulty loving yourself and receiving love and support
* Feeling of victimization and subsequent resentment
* Difficulty forgiving others
* Inability to give and receive love easily
* Feeling of isolation

Imbalanced Heart and Shoulders in Action

Meghan came to me because she wanted to get rid of the knots in her shoulders. Although she was only in her late thirties, she could feel her body beginning to hunch over and tighten up. On our first consultation, Meghan also shared that she was grappling with anxiety, depression, and fear.

Meghan thought I was psychic when I asked her if she was dealing with heartbreak. In actuality, she was exhibiting common symptoms I see all the time in clients who are closed off to love. In her case, these symptoms included tight shoulders and a compressed upper body, which both stem from the fact that we begin to physically cave in and collapse in the heart area when we experience heartbreak. Most of us are totally unaware we are doing this. I don't think Meghan even realized how closed off she'd become until we began to talk through her situation. She was one of those people who gave a ton but didn't know how to receive in turn.

Meghan and I worked on opening up the front of her shoulders, chest, and collarbones through movement medicine, emotional hygiene, breathwork, and self-massage. We cleared out a lot of the physical density and emotional energy that had built up in her system, like dried-up and brittle fascia that had turned into scar tissue, and knots that were literally gluing her into a compressed, thick, stuck posture. This posture was pulling Meghan forward and making her look and feel defeated, depressed, and hunched. We also got to the root cause of the clutching in her shoulders and alleviated density in her upper back so that the back of her shoulders weren't constantly tense and feeling as if they were being pulled forward. As a result of no longer having to compensate for her shoulders,

Meghan was able to reconnect to her core. Together, we were able to get Meghan's body into a more upright and open posture, which made her feel calmer and more at ease. Meghan told me it felt as if the weight of the world had melted off her shoulders, and people were responding to her in a more positive way.

Within a couple of months, Meghan was noticeably more uplifted and upright. There was less tension in her middle back. She felt more open to the world and more present. From this more calm and connected state, we were able to bring some aware-ness to what Meghan was holding in her body on an emotional level. We worked on letting go of some heartbreak from her past, reframing it as a lesson rather than a victimization. This, in turn, allowed Meghan to release some guilt she'd been carrying around from her childhood. She opened up to self-love and, from there, learned to receive love as well.

Meghan's anxiety dissipated, as did her depression. Together, we worked on an exercise that I call "The List," which I'll share later on in this chapter: Meghan wrote out a specific list describ-ing the partner she wanted to manifest in her life to match who she had evolved into. I'm happy to tell you that he arrived a few months later. Meghan is now married, with two kids, to her ideal match, with whom she feels free to both give and receive.

Get to Know Your Heart and Shoulders

We will now concentrate on creating freedom in the heart and shoulders, as well as unwinding, rebalancing, and restoring this power center. This will build upon what you already know about lifting your body up from the upper core.

The heart and shoulders power center extends from the upper rib cage to the base of the neck, and includes your shoulders, chest, collar bones, upper back, and heart area.

So many of us have tight and knotted-up shoulders, whether it's the result of injury, technology, logistics, a broken heart, resentment, or an energy blockage. Our shoulders become congested from hunching over our computers, clinging or gripping to stressors, and shrinking ourselves down, to name just a few common causes. When our shoulders are chronically tight, our fascia can effectively glue the shoulders forward. We call shoulders in this position *protracted*.

When our shoulders are protracted, it causes our chest to cave in. The shoulders compensate by becoming what I call "long-tight." This makes them weak, vulnerable, and glued into that forward position. The shoulder fascia and muscles are stretched farther than they should be in order to compensate for congestion in the chest.

When we are angry we tend to squeeze our arms into our body, which tightens up everything in the shoulder area. Most of us don't even realize we're doing this. Anger generally comes from the desire to control something and a feeling that we have somehow been wrong or slighted. Clutching our arms in like this is a physical manifestation of this emotion and desire to control. While the feeling may be totally legitimate, we don't want it to stagnate within us and weigh us down.

When we think of expressive parts of the body, we generally tend to think of facial features, such as the eyes, brow, or mouth. I find that the shoulders are also incredibly expressive and telling. Different positions of the shoulders can reveal different mindsets. For instance, raised shoulders reveal fear and the resultant anger. Rounded shoulders reveal that someone is overburdened with the demands of life or is taking on more responsibility than they can handle. Overly retracted and pulled-back shoulders have to do with holding back emotions, pushing through, and trying to force things to happen.

When a person becomes angry, they feel a strong wave of energy. Part of the anger reaction is a rush of adrenaline, which causes the cardiac and respiratory rhythms to accelerate and the voluntary muscles to receive more energy due to the glycogen liberated by the liver. This manifests as the feeling of a strong need to express anger through words and action. When anger is repressed, energy is concentrated and trapped in the upper armpits, shoulders, and neck. It can also compress the lymph nodes and make them sluggish.

The Lymphatic System

I like to think of the lymphatic system as the garbage disposal of the body. It is responsible for removing waste and toxins. In this polluted world, the lymphatic system is more important than ever before. We are exposed to thousands of toxins daily, including household cleaning products, beauty products, processed foods, plastics, chemically based foods, and other environmental toxins. This elimination is incredibly important for immunity, optimal health, and even weight loss.

The lymphatic system flushes out inflammation, toxins, and even blocked energy. The actual lymph nodes—which power the system—live around our armpits. When our lymph nodes are blocked, the lymphatic system can't do its job. We want to prevent this from happening, because when the lymphatic system is blocked, our entire body is blocked as a result, and it hangs on to all of those things we want to expunge, both physically and energetically. Since toxicity can play a huge role in premature aging and losing or keeping excess weight off, this system must be cleared when we are seeking optimal health. The movement medicine and foods in this chapter will help you do exactly that.

The Heart and Shoulders and Holistic Health

In acupuncture, one of the anxiety pressure points is found in this power center, right around the breastbone. This area can become energetically blocked with emotions like envy, hate, bitterness, resentment, anger, and feeling inadequate. This emotional buildup of negative stuck energy can literally lead to a tight chest, a defeated posture, possibly depression, inability to take a deep breath, an overwhelming feeling of stress, and even an anxiety attack.

Because we hold so many of our emotions in our physical bodies, we can wind up marinating in them without even realizing it. Sometimes these negative emotions are the result of our own experience; other times, we carry them for others; and, sometimes, it's a combination of both. It's good to feel these emotions, bring them to the surface, and let them move through. When we carry our heavy emotions through life with us, we begin reacting to them, which can infuse our relationships with a stubborn or vindictive quality.

Now, this isn't to say that we won't all experience troubles, heartbreaks, betrayals, or some measure of resentment in our lives. Of course we will! That's part of the human experience. If we never experience any of these darker aspects, it probably indicates the far bigger problem that we're not connecting with others in the first place. We don't want that either. But we *do* want to find a coping mechanism for navigating and releasing these tougher emotions when they arise, rather than clinging to and collecting them to the point where we can't connect at all. To heal, we need to allow ourselves to feel emotions, move them through our bodies and learn from them, then release them. And we need to practice all three of these things on a regular basis.

We all wear our stories. The next time you walk down a street, see if you can identify people who are hunched forward from the weight of dealing with heartbreak. Now see if you can identify those with open, optimistic hearts and relaxed shoulders. Identifying these qualities has little to do with intuition—it's based on body language and breath. I bet you'll find it easy to spot.

I use this skill in my practice daily and it provides so much insight into my clients. I can then use the information I observe to offer my clients awareness about simple shifts in their lives that can create a huge impact. It might be as simple as saying, "You look a little bit defeated. Are you running up against any walls in your life?" Often, once a client puts voice to this, they allow themselves to feel the emotion, which takes the power out of the situation and its impact on their physical, emotional, and mental state. The body tells the story of our lives. Once we become aware about the ways in which our body is compensating for misalignment, rigidity, and dis-ease and become attuned to our own repressed emotional energy, we have the ability to become free in a split second.

When we accumulate negative feelings that result from our interactions—or lack thereof—with others, we hold ourselves differently. The weight of this isolation weighs us down. We hunch over, our head juts forward, our chest caves in, our collarbones roll down, and gravity compresses us. We might also hold our weight too far forward in our feet or walk around with our shoulders in our ears, both of which make it difficult to feel grounded. Now, not only are we holding more weight than we need to, but we also don't feel like we have a strong base. Since the thoracic-lumbar connection is found at the base of our shoulder blades, anything that impacts our shoulders also impacts our head. This means that what we experience in the heart and shoulders literally impacts us all the way up and down our body, from the bottoms of our feet up to the top of our head.

The Heart Chakra

The heart chakra, found in the chest and shoulder area, is associated with the color green and the element of air. When it is healthy, energy can flow into and out of the heart chakra with ease, much like air does. This chakra overlaps the thymus gland, which regulates our immune system. Author Caroline Myss explains in her book *Anatomy of the Spirit*, "Unquestionably, a strong link exists between physical and emotional stresses and specific illnesses. This connection has been well-documented, for instance, with regard to heart disease and hypertension and the so-called Type A personality. My particular insights, however, have shown me that emotional *and spiritual* stresses and dis-eases are the root causes of *all* physical illnesses."

The heart chakra deals with matters of forgiveness and acceptance. These are equally important in our relationships with others and our relationship with ourselves. To exercise both forgiveness and acceptance, we need to tap into compassion. Our heart chakra offers us the ability to exercise connecting from a place of compassion—with ourselves, our loved ones, and the world.

As is the case with the shoulders, when our heart chakra is open, we feel more connected and fulfilled. We are able to participate in a healthy exchange of energy within our relationships. Perhaps you've noticed that when you are dealing with heartbreak, you subconsciously hold in emotion. This is a function of protection, but it prevents any energy exchange from happening. When we are in this state, we cannot give or receive in a balanced, healthy, fulfilling way. We get stuck.

When we find balance in the heart, it's much easier to see the beauty in everything—and to feel it, too. We can create deep and meaningful relationships that offer us freedom rather than tethering us down. We can connect and relate, give and receive. It also allows us to exercise love, gratitude, and acceptance in everything we do. This applies not just to romantic love, but to love in all of its glorious forms, big and small.

When the heart chakra is blocked or imbalanced, it can lead to jealousy, codependency, or withdrawal. We bring negativity we have acquired from past situations into new relationships and connections. When we achieve balance in the heart, we can instead see people and experiences with clarity and deal with them with compassion, love, and—just as importantly—discernment.

The Heart, Shoulders, and the Pelvic Floor Connection

Do you remember the story I told about the woman I met at a dinner party whose shoulders immediately melted when she released stress through her pelvic floor by doing a Kegel? This is because the shoulders and jaw are a mirror of the pelvic floor. Nine times out of ten, when our pelvic floor is relaxed and de-stressed, so are our shoulders. The opposite is also true: if you can release clutching in your pelvic floor, you can release a huge amount of tension from your shoulders.

As a result of tightness in the pelvic floor, many people have developed the habit of holding themselves upright in a manner that involves subconsciously clutching their shoulders—sometimes all the way up toward their ears. This is actually a natural biological reaction of fear and protection that we have carried over from our hunter and gatherer ancestors. The difference is that our forebears naturally released this stance once danger passed. When we lift our shoulders up toward our ears, our arms rotate inward and forward, which has a direct impact on the shoulder and chest area. The gravitational force constantly pulling us forward causes our heart to cave and creates knots in our shoulder blades. The energy in our heart and shoulders begins to grip and stagnate. Beyond the physical manifestation, this energetically translates to a lodging of emotions in the heart area. Once this happens, we can become stuck—energy is blocked from coming in and going out. With this, we also lock stress and emotion into these tissues. Today, we can stay frozen here on a near-constant basis, our bodies tightening up, especially in our ever-so-malleable connective tissues. We live with a subconscious physical bearing down that sends a message to our nervous system that we are in danger or in survival mode. To create length, we want to ground our feet down to the earth and gracefully lift our head and spine, letting our shoulders stay low and relaxed.

Many people try to release this feeling of stress in their chest or shoulders by practicing the opposite of this crunching-up motion. They attempt to correct by shoving their shoulders down tightly all the time. (Type A doers are especially prone to this movement. It's an offshoot of trying to "do" their way out of every situation, including stress. Obviously, this is counterproductive.) Because this motion isn't natural either, it only results in another form of locking and force, and also creates unwanted tension. You can roll out your shoulders and get massaged to your heart's content, but until you learn to unlock your pelvic floor and calm your nervous system, you will never be able to truly work out the deep tension in your shoulders. You will continue to hold internalized stress, tension, and emotional scar tissue there.

We want to find balance to alleviate the stress that roots itself in the pelvic floor and travels up to the neck. At least once a day, practice releasing your pelvic floor, remaining acutely aware of how your shoulders react. (See pages 36–37 for instructions on releasing the pelvic floor.)

The Shoulders and Heart Stress Connection

Even though the stress and emotional weight we carry on our shoulders may be symbolic, it feels very real to our bodies and affects us in measurable and quantifiable ways. There are two types of stress: the pressure of our daily life and to-do lists, and the other deeper and sometimes unresolved trauma of emotional stress and buried feelings. Both weigh us down.

We live our lives in go-go-go mode, not bothering to stop and take note of how we feel. Even when we're not in motion, we're still not taking the time for personal inventory—we're checking our phones or on social media or ruminating on what we need to do next or should have done differently. While it's true that we all have a lot to do, we also tend to put a lot of self-imposed pressure upon ourselves, like we're hassled by our own busy lives. When we're under pressure, we tend to become unfocused and less efficient. This creates even more stress.

Stress and pressure aren't going away, so we've got to evolve into a place where each of us takes responsibility for actively managing the impact we have on our own lives. We must start choosing to make ourselves, our health, our time, and our relationships a priority. We need to expand our mind, thoughts, and belief system so we don't get broken down by a too-connected, too-active life. Circumstances will always be up and down, so it's critical that we train ourselves to take moments to breathe, be present, and be mindful of the right here, right now. Learning how to create these moments of focus can help us dramatically change our reactions and relax into the life we are living

Emotional stress can come in a variety of ways, but, as it relates to this area of the body, stress tends to result from resentment, frustration, fear, and jealousy. Holding on to these emotions causes us tension, disease, and dis-ease.

While many of us may not have the innate ability to detect the state of our pelvic floor, deep core, or diaphragm without some practice, almost all of us can tell when we're holding stress and tension in our shoulders. The good news is that once we identify it, we can resolve it by treating the underlying causes! We can take inventory and evaluate the top stressors in our lives. We can do the physical and mental work of caring for the different stress containers in the body. Once we understand this, we can create more organization and less hassle to enjoy and flow gracefully through our lives.

When it comes to stress in this area of the body, we want to pause in the moment and choose to harness the energy rather than responding with the gripping reaction that uses so much of our precious energy. We can actually make this stress work for us by learning to adapt and channel stress into arousal and motivation. We can remember that we are not in a life-or-death situation, so we can let go of our survival reaction. We can take a measured look at our circumstances, reprioritize, take responsibility for the decisions we're making with our time, shift to a state of gratitude, and release the residue of resentment so that it does not build up.

HEART AND SHOULDERS STRESS HYGIENE

To begin building new, nonreactive habits around stress, try this simple stress-combating exercise the next time you catch yourself in a moment of clutching.

Allow your feet to feel grounded and your arms to hang down. Imagine you have 10-pound weights on your elbows so the weight of your shoulders is not being held up by your neck. Let your shoulder blades gently relax downward. Take an inhale and draw your shoulder blades up to your ears; exhale as you roll your shoulders down. Continue this movement for 10 full rounds of breath. End by shaking your arms out to release any remaining tension in the upper-arm area and focus on something you're grateful for.

Movement Medicine for the Heart and Shoulders

Give Yourself a Hug

Lie down on the mat face-up and place the ball between the tops of your shoulder blades so that it is supporting your neck at the base of your skull. Inhale as you cross your arms to give yourself a hug, and wrap your fingers around your shoulder blades. Inhale as you reach your arms wide with your palms facing up, allowing your chest to expand. Exhale as you cross your arms again, this time with the opposite arm on top. Bring your fingers to your shoulder blades and massage the upper middle back to create space in your chest. Repeat this series of movements 8 times.

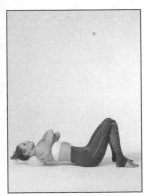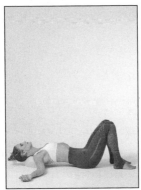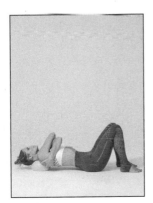

Give Yourself a Hug

Front of Shoulder Roll

Lie face-down on the mat and place the ball under the front of your left shoulder. Extend your left arm out to the side. Bend your right arm, with your elbow facing out to the side. Line your right thumb up with your armpit and face your fingertips forward. Inhale as you press down into your right palm and turn to look over your right shoulder, twisting your head and ribs to the right, and reaching your left arm long to the left to open up your left shoulder. Inhale and return to center. Repeat this series of movements 8 times on each side.

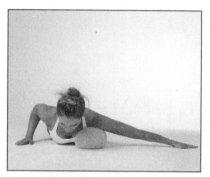 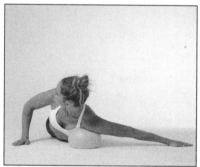

Front of Shoulder Roll

Rotator Cuff Alignment

Place the ball under the front of your left shoulder. Bring your right forearm to the mat and rest your forehead on your right hand. Bring the top of your left hand to rest on your lower back. Allow your left elbow to drape down toward the mat. Keeping the top of your left hand on your lower back, inhale as you reach your elbow up. Exhale as you slowly slide your elbow down as close to the floor as possible. Repeat this series of movements 8 times.

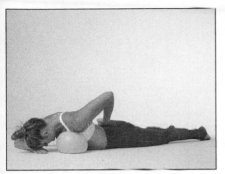
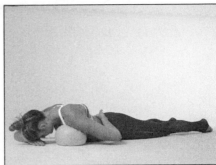

Rotator Cuff Alignment

Airplane Arm

Place the ball under the front of your left shoulder. Place your right palm down with your thumb lined up with your right shoulder, with your elbow bent. Reach your left arm long so that you are reaching toward your left pinky toe with your palms facing up. Relax the top of your shoulders. Inhale as you reach your left arm out to the side. Exhale as you reach your arm out and down toward your hip. Repeat this series of movements 8 times on each side.

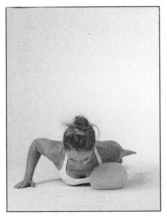
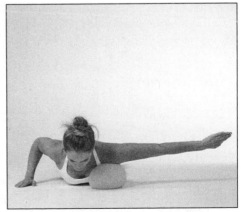

Airplane Arm

Heart Release with Swan Stretch

Lie face-down on the mat and place the ball underneath your breast bone, with your hips down on the mat and legs long behind you. Place your palms down and line your thumbs up with your armpits, elbows reaching back. Inhale as you extend your spine and lift your heart, opening your chest. Exhale as you round down, letting the ball roll up through your heart and chest area. Repeat this series of movements 8 times.

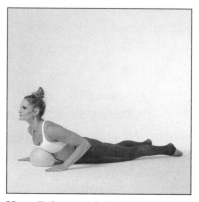 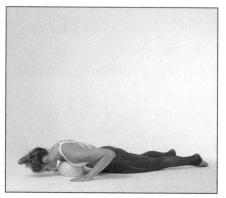

Heart Release with Swan Stretch

Heart Opening Bow

Lie face-down on the mat and place the ball under your breast bone. Bend your knees and reach your arms back so that your palms are holding on to the tops of your feet. Inhale as you lift your heart, kicking your feet into your hands and activating your hamstrings. Exhale as you come back down. Release your legs and arms down to the ground. Inhale and reach your right foot out to the right. Exhale and reach your left foot out to the left, fully stretching your heart and shoulders. Repeat this series of movements 8 times.

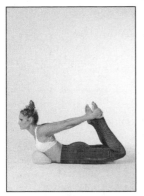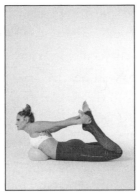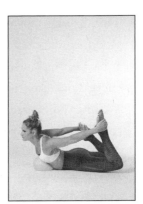

Heart Opening Bow

Chest Melt with Sway

Lie face-down on the mat and place the ball on the front of your left shoulder below your collarbones. Bend your elbows out to the side and place your palms on the floor. Inhale and sway your body to the right, allowing the ball to massage your left shoulder. Exhale and come to the center of your chest. Move the ball to the other side and repeat this series of movements 8 times on each side.

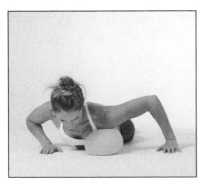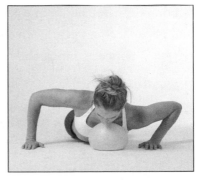

Chest Melt with Sway

Heart-Focused Breathing

This breath will open and soften your heart, oxygenate your blood, and flood your body and mind with fresh energy. Do this as part of your movement medicine or any time you want to bring energy and attention to your heart.

Shift your awareness to your heart area. As you breathe in for a count of 6, release your pelvic floor and feel gratitude fill your heart. As you exhale, think of someone or something you deeply appreciate and send your heart energy to them. Repeat this expansive pattern of inhaling and exhaling love for 10 full rounds of breath. Try this when you're stuck in traffic or washing the dishes, and feel the shift.

Heal and Balance Your Shoulders and Heart

Get a Fresh Breath of Air

The heart loves air. Get your heart energy flowing and bring yourself into the moment by taking some nice, hearty inhales of fresh air. That might mean going outside or just opening up the windows of your house and letting the air filter in. Be present and grounded and give yourself the *experience* of nutrient-dense oxygen—notice its smells and how it feels on your skin.

Make a Practice of Forgiveness . . .

We often think of forgiveness as something that requires action— or, more specifically, *interaction*. However, this doesn't account for unfinished business that we might have with people who are gone, who we choose to no longer interact with, or with whom a conversation about the topic at hand may not be possible for any number of other reasons. But what's important to remember is that forgiving others is about letting go of the burden of anger, hurt, frustration, fear, or other negative emotions. At the end of the day, forgiveness is all about you, and you can take care of it *right now*. There is no need to hold on to resentment for a single second longer; it actually only harms you and the holding doesn't change the outcome.

We talk about cultivating a practice of gratitude all of the time. This is important—but what about forgiveness? It is just as important, if not more so. Make an exercise of practicing forgiveness not only of others, but also of yourself.

Write down three things you're holding on to or feeling resentful about in your journal. Think about what might help you resolve those feelings—what would take away some of the power that the source of conflict has over you? Logically think through what a resolution would look like and feel like, and put it in writing. Then, again in writing, explore the freedom of letting go of the pain, and to take the healing even further, you can even try turning your pain into purpose.

... and Shift into a State of Gratitude, Too

With our heart clear of resentment, there is room for forgiveness. We can now practice gratitude in a more powerful way than ever before.

Of course, gratitude can be incorporated into life as a practice in any number of ways; you should do whatever resonates most with you. However, I like to do this simple ritual: over dinner every night, every person at the table shares three things they are grateful for. The trick is, you can never repeat the same thing.

You will soon find that this seemingly small practice of gratitude allows you to see and connect with the world in new ways. Consciously or subconsciously, you will be on the lookout each day for the three things you are grateful for. It brings you into the moment and makes you more aware of all there is to be grateful for. Soon you'll find that it's difficult to limit your list to just three objects of gratitude per day and you will realize how blessed you already are.

Learn to Love Unconditionally—Beginning with You

Make a regular habit of becoming specifically aware of and accountable for your own feelings. This can start with small actions that net big results. Say no to things you are uncomfortable with or that don't feel right. Ask for things you desire. I often say, "The answer is always no unless you ask." Establish boundaries in your personal and professional life. Keep at it, even if it feels difficult at first. That's okay. As you practice more and more, it will become easier and easier, until it finally becomes innate.

The more you are able to nurture your heart, the more you can open it to give and receive love, the more you can cultivate awareness of it and what it needs, and the more wholeheartedly you will be able to interact with others and truly fall in love with yourself and your life.

Build Your Dream Partner

When we think of the heart, we think of love. And when we think of love, we often first think of romantic love. While romantic relationships are far from the *only* kind of love the heart deals with, they are also something most of us want.

Be intentional about who you draw into your life and your heart. Write down the super-specific qualities you want in your ideal partner. This is not about a fairytale. It's about connecting with your true self and what your inner being really desires, rather than defaulting to what others think you need or emulating what you see in the media or on Instagram. This is about the real you, and you've got to define it to align with it. This is about accountability and compatibility. It's also about integrating your mind and thoughts with your emotions and feelings. Through this exercise, you will align your intentions with your actions and learn how to be the partner you want to be with.

Don't limit yourself—allow your deepest, truest authentic desires to surface. It can be harder than we think to actually identify these qualities in a truly resonant way. Focus on the personality traits you need in a partner, rather than the superficial physicality of them, which fades so quickly. When I wrote my list, some of the descriptors I used were: *loyal, loving, interested in spiritualty, family-oriented, strong, sense of humor, open-minded, athletic, adventurous, honest, trustworthy, dependable, charismatic, kind, passionate, loves to travel, and handy.*

Take some time with this and continue adding to the list over time. Give your subconscious desires a chance to rise to the surface. This is an exercise in trusting yourself, your instincts, and your intuitive understanding of the path that is meant for you. In doing this, you plant a seed and send a message to the quantum field. When you have finished, put your list in a drawer and surrender to knowing that it's yours. Don't cling to it.

My best guess is that the next time you find it, you'll be shocked at how much closer—or on the nose!—to this dream partner you've come.

TAKE A GODDESS-OF-LOVE BATH

This soothing and detoxifying blend can feel especially indulgent when dealing with inflammation, or when you're looking to soothe the skin and lock in moisture. You will emerge from this bath feeling and looking like the goddess you are.

To prepare, enclose equal amounts of up to 6 tablespoons each of the following herbs and minerals in a muslin drawstring bag or double layer of cheesecloth (after you've tried it once, feel free to adjust the amounts of each ingredient to your liking):

Calendula
Lavender
Magnesium chloride salt
Oats
Rose petals

Hang the bag on the faucet and turn the water on. As the tub fills, the water will run through the herbs, infusing the water with healing herbal power.

Mantra and Visualization for the Shoulders

---

*"It is safe for me to be vulnerable and allow myself the giving
and receiving of love effortlessly and unconditionally."*

Find a comfortable seated position on a cushion, roller, or squishy
ball. Crisscross your legs and allow your hips to relax. Drop
down into awareness of your pelvic floor, allowing yourself to
feel grounded, light, and spacious. Find a place of relaxation and
surrender.

In everyday life, the shoulders tend to shift up toward the ears,
whether it's from hunching over, sitting too much, or the busy
ness or stress of life. This constant holding pattern makes it difficult to let go of built-up tightness and compression.

All of this begins in the nervous system and how we react and
respond to life. By connecting the pelvic floor to the shoulder
area, we gain the ability to let go and turn the stress button off.
With that comes a sense of ease, calm, and grace. We are going to
use the pelvic floor to help our shoulders relax.

Feel your shoulder blades calmly melting down toward your
back pockets. Don't force this, just allow. Feel the openness in
your heart and the space between each of your vertebrae. Notice
how effortless it feels to sit in gravity: when you allow your sitz
bones to act as the foundation of your spine, you feel effortlessly
supported without having to hold yourself up from your shoulders. As you notice this support and stability, allow your shoulders to relax even more. Imagine you have 10-pound weights on

your elbows, and feel your elbows drop down. Notice the space it creates between your ears and your shoulders.

Bring your awareness back to your pelvic floor. Contract your pelvic floor, pulling it up and in as if you were pulling a rosebud into your body with a suction cup. Now, slowly feel the contrast as you allow the pelvic floor to open and expand, blooming like a flower. Use this sense of contrasting feelings to begin to connect with the idea of letting go. As you repeat this contraction and expansion, notice how your pelvic floor affects your deep core and then your chest.

Shift your attention to your heart area. Notice if you're holding an emotion—a resentment, a fear, a jealousy, or anxiety. Whatever emotion you feel, notice it, acknowledge it, and then imagine yourself blowing it away to the heavens. Release it. Exhale as you feel yourself soften. Notice if you have a sensation of weight on your shoulders. Complete the same exercise, looking at the emotion or situation that rests there, acknowledging it and blowing it away.

Imagine the space that you have now created for deeper self-love, deeper receiving of love, and deeper giving of love. Feel a white light shining out of your heart area. Think about the people you love. Shine that light directly to their heart. Feel that love coming back to you from them. Notice how it softens you, how it alleviates anxiety, fear, and depression, how it allows you to connect to the deeper inner-knowing of you.

With softness comes strength and power—the beautiful, elegant power of openness and flow, and the power of connection and love. Love is the greatest superpower on the planet. Love is light. Love shines light over the darkness.

Inhale, filling up your lungs. Exhale, letting it all go as you melt your shoulders down.

Activate Your Love Superpower Through the Heart and Shoulders

When our shoulders and chest tighten up, it can lock our energy. When this happens, it's harder to give and receive love—plain and simple. The good stuff can't get in, and the bad stuff can't get out.

A common scenario looks something like this: someone experiences upsetting treatment in a relationship but doesn't express their feelings. Because they are not expunging that energy by putting voice to it, the emotion becomes locked in their body. Remember, the lymph nodes love to expunge—that's what they were built for. When this doesn't happen, blockage occurs. In this case, that blockage is the result of stagnant resentment.

Most of us have the tendency to subconsciously squeeze our upper arms into our body and clutch them there or bear down, either out of frustration or as a defense mechanism. Thus, we see the action of clutching rather than releasing resentment here in the upper chest area.

Locked-in resentment extends to the breasts as well. It's no mistake that breast cancer is one of the top diseases of women in the Western world. Since my mom died of breast cancer, work in this area is particularly near and dear to my heart. Conjure up an image of the archetypical female martyr, who bears the weight of her loved ones on her shoulders and always puts herself last. She is so weighed down by this that it ultimately hunches her over and closes her heart. As born nurturers, women often have a difficult time receiving. In so many ways, this comes from a beautifully giving and empathetic place. However, when we do this at the expense of filling up our own cup, it can become detrimental—not only emotionally, but also physically. In its most extreme form, this behavior can manifest itself in a disease like breast cancer, which is, not coincidentally, found in our heart center. The great news is that we have the power to shift our attention back to ourselves in healthy ways that may help prevent and cure.

Now let's conjure up a different image. Think about the weight of others you bear in your own life. Notice if you can feel the burden of that in your shoulders. Do they feel locked or tied down? Now imagine that you can free yourself from that weight, while still living from a place of love, compassion, and forgiveness. Really imagine what that would look like in action. Can you feel a slight shift and relaxation in your shoulders? Do you feel a bit lighter just thinking about what life would look like if your body existed in this energy and you lived and interacted from that place?

It is with the combination of these qualities of love, compassion, and forgiveness that we prevent resentment from getting stuck and settling in. So often—especially in women—that feeling of a closed-off heart and weighted-down shoulders results in a feeling of disconnection, from both others and ourselves. When we create time for ourselves and free ourselves of resentment and the burden that comes with it, we create more room to expand our heart, physically and emotionally.

To connect with others in a truly meaningful way, we must choose to live in a state of love and feeling connected to all beings. In addition, we must choose to not just give, but also receive—and receive love from ourselves, too. We can give to a point that we no longer have the ability to receive. Instead, we effectively close ourselves off. By bringing awareness to and healing to this part of the body, we can learn to open up and connect in a way that flows and does not leave behind a residue of stagnation and blockage.

The best gift we can offer to the world is to love ourselves, love our families, practice gratitude, and live in the present moment.

ALTERNATIVE THERAPIES FOR THE HEART AND SHOULDERS

Aromatherapy

Jasmine

Warm, rich, floral, and sweet, jasmine symbolizes hope, happiness, and love in many different spiritual traditions. Some think that when diffused or applied topically, the scent can promote optimism. In the heart area, jasmine is particularly healing when it comes to relationships and the wounds they leave behind. Its uplifting fragrance opens the heart chakra to love and compassion.

Palo Santo

Palo santo is a type of tree that has been used for centuries by indigenous people of the Andes for spiritual purification and energy cleansing. Palo santo comes in stick form and is burned much like incense.

Palo santo cleans negative energy and restores tranquility and calm in our body and environment. It invites in love, creativity, and good fortune. Its scent promotes feelings of joy, enhances clarity and concentration, and reduces stress.

Crystals

All of these crystals will help to open space for both giving and receiving more love. They are also known for their ability to assist with alleviating and releasing resentment.

- **Emerald**—enhances unity, unconditional love, and partnerships; opens the heart
- **Jade**—harmonizes the heart, releases emotions, and symbolizes purity and serenity
- **Rose quartz**—attracts love, brings unconditional love and infinite peace, and purifies and opens the heart

To heal your heart, select the crystal that resonates with you most and place it in the center of your chest. As it rests there, meditate, relax, or visualize the outcome you hope to receive. For a more consistent infusion of healing vibes, you can also carry your selected crystal with you in your purse or pocket, wear it as jewelry, or place it in your home or car.

Tea

Tulsi, also known as holy basil, is the most sacred herb in India. This heart-healthy tea packs in a lot of magnesium, which helps prevent heart disease by helping the blood vessels work properly. It promotes the free flow of blood and includes antioxidants that protect the heart from free radical damage. Regularly drinking tulsi tea can reduce cholesterol levels and lower blood pressure.

As if this wasn't enough, tulsi also helps maintain normal cortisol levels, which means less stress. It also delays signs of aging and promotes beautiful, healthy skin. Just one mug of tulsi tea a day can leave you both feeling and looking beautiful. I love Organic India Tulsi Tea Original, which can be found on Amazon.

Nourish Your Shoulders and Heart

Herbs for the Heart and Shoulders: Gardenia

Gardenia is known as "the happiness herb." It is believed that this flower will attract love into your life. Not only that, but its beautiful fragrance is very calming to the heart. Place a fresh gardenia in a small bowl of water and allow yourself to be intoxicated by its heart-healing scent.

Minerals for the Heart and Shoulders: Dark Chocolate

It seems fitting for the heart center that we get our minerals in the form of...chocolate! Dark chocolate, to be exact. Experts have found that chocolate is good for the heart, circulation, and brain. Dark chocolate is loaded with minerals that positively impact your health, such as potassium, calcium, magnesium, and iron. Made from the seed of the cocoa tree, dark chocolate is one of the best sources of antioxidants on the planet. Dark chocolate also boosts serotonin and endorphin levels, relieves pain, and is a mood booster.

But wait, there's more! Urologists from San Raffaele Hospital in Milan, Italy, questioned 163 women about their consumption of chocolate and sexual fulfillment. They found that women who had a daily intake of chocolate showed higher levels of desire than women who did not. Yes, please!

FOODS THAT HEAL THE HEART AND SHOULDERS

- **Leafy greens**—arugula, bok choy, collards, dandelion greens, kale, mustard greens, romaine, spinach, and sprouts
- **Omega 3s**—cold-water oily fish like anchovies, herring, mackerel, salmon, and sardines
- **Green-colored foods**—avocados, celery, green apples, green peppers, kiwi, pears, squash, watercress, and zucchini

Love Elixir

MAKES 16 OUNCES

This gorgeous and beautifying pink-hued drink will fill your heart with love and passion. Hibiscus is high in vitamin C and antioxidants. It is also known to help regulate blood pressure, according to the American Heart Association. Rosewater is thought to support the heart, inviting in more love and openness. It helps enhance mood and relieve depression and stress. As if that's not enough, rosewater also contains anti-inflammatory and antioxidant properties that help reduce skin redness and puffiness, and protect cells from damage. It's almost as if it was straight from the fountain of youth!

  16 ounces alkaline or filtered water
  1 cup dried hibiscus flowers
  1 cup raspberries (fresh or frozen)
  Juice of 1 lemon
  2 tablespoons rosewater
  1 ½ teaspoons raw honey (optional)

Bring the water to boil in a small saucepan. Place the hibiscus and raspberries in a jug or large glass jar. Once the water has boiled, add it to the jar and let it brew for at least an hour. Strain the water through a sieve into a jug. Next, add the lemon juice, rosewater, and honey if desired.

Store remaining elixir in the fridge for up to 1 week.

Green Goddess Tonic

MAKES 8 OUNCES

1 green apple, chopped
2 ribs celery, cut into 3-inch lengths
Juice of a fresh lemon
½ bunch parsley, with stems

Combine the apple, celery, lemon, and parsley in a juicer and blend until you have achieved a juice consistency. Enjoy!

Heart-Healing Veggie Broth

MAKES 6 QUARTS

This nourishing vegetable broth is bursting with healing love for your heart and coziness to relax your shoulders and open your heart. It's like consuming your whole veggie garden in the form of a hug. Not only does this broth taste delicious, but it also supports the immune system. Vegetable broth is naturally loaded with essential nutrients to support immunity, along with whole-food sources of zinc, vitamin B12, and calcium. Zinc is an essential mineral for assisting immune system function and also contributes to protecting cells from free radicals. Vitamin B12 helps reduce fatigue, while also supporting immunity.

If you've never heard of kombu, it is a mineral-rich seaweed that adds a savory flavor to stocks and broths. Kombu is usually found in the Asian section of a grocery store.

6 unpeeled carrots, cut into thirds	2 unpeeled sweet potatoes, quartered
2 unpeeled yellow onions, cut into chunks	5 unpeeled cloves garlic, halved
1 leek, white and green parts, cut into thirds	½ bunch fresh parsley
	1 (8-inch) strip of kombu seaweed
1 bunch celery, including the heart, cut into thirds	12 black peppercorns
	2 bay leaves
4 unpeeled red potatoes, quartered	8 quarts cold, filtered water
	1 teaspoon sea salt

Rinse all of the vegetables well, including the kombu. In a 12-quart or larger stockpot, combine the carrots, onions, leek, celery, potatoes, sweet potatoes, garlic, parsley, kombu, peppercorns, and bay leaves. Fill the pot with the water just below the rim, cover, and bring to a boil.

Remove the lid, lower the heat, and simmer, uncovered, for 2 hours. Add more water if the veggies start to peek out of the pot. Simmer until you can taste the full richness of the veggies.

Strain the broth through a large strainer, then add salt to taste.

To store, allow the broth to cool to room temperature before refrigerating or freezing. Store in an airtight container in the refrigerator for 5 to 7 days or in the freezer for up to 4 months.

7

The Head Power Center: Connection Superpower

SIGNS YOUR HEAD NEEDS SOME LOVE

Physical

* Clenched jaw
* Forward head posture
* Furrowed brow and wrinkled forehead
* Frowning mouth
* Saggy jowls
* Tight, stiff, short, or weak neck

* Bags under your eyes or sunken eyes
* Regular headaches and/or migraines
* Ringing in ears
* Frequent sinus infections or sore throats
* Disconnected to your body

Emotional

* Swallowing emotions
* Difficulty seeing things clearly
* Lack of imagination
* Self-loathing thoughts
* Disconnected from emotions
* Feeling separate and disconnected from others
* Feeling better than others
* Judgmental feelings toward self and others

* Overthinking and overprocessing
* Misalignment of thoughts, words, and actions
* Inability to keep promises
* Difficulty communicating feelings
* Lack of a feeling of connection with something bigger than yourself

The Imbalanced Head in Action

When I met Barbara, her head was hunched forward, her jaw was locked, her neck was tight, and her shoulders were rounded forward. Her fascia was incredibly brittle. In general, she looked defeated. Whenever clients come to me in this state, it's usually a sign that they are stuck in a state of flight-or-flight, and that their cerebrospinal fluid is blocked and stagnant, which throws the nervous system into distress. At first, Barbara and I didn't talk about what was going on in her life. We just got moving and help ing her reconnect to her body again.

Clients experiencing the sort of head and neck issues that Barbara had usually fall at one of two opposite extremes of the spectrum. They are either in a lot of pain, or totally disconnected and numb. Barbara was in pain. Constantly. All of the tightness was getting to her, and she was also experiencing migraines. We used awareness, breathwork, and establishing a connection with her pelvic floor to start reawakening Barbara's system. Then we began using the squishy ball to cradle her head and help reestab-lish a normal range of motion in the area in a gentle, restorative way. With this, we created more space and allowed her locked tissue to begin to rehydrate and her joints to become more mobile.

Over time, Barbara's head moved back into alignment so that it floated above her spine rather than hunching forward. Her face relaxed and her wrinkles softened—the effect was almost like natural Botox. Her jaw released. She looked more radiant and had a new glow to her. People began to ask Barbara what had changed. What was she doing, and could they do it too?

It wasn't until Barbara found physical alignment that she

began to share with me what had been going on in her life. Her husband had been cheating on her for quite some time. Rather than putting voice to how this made her feel, Barbara got stuck in her head about the situation and lodged everything inside. She ruminated on all of the reasons why she had caused this violation to occur. She blamed herself for her husband's transgressions with the narrative that she was not good enough.

As Barbara's head came into alignment, she found her voice and started expressing and releasing her swallowed emotions. She told me what had happened and how she had been hurting. Her brain began to work in a new, bigger-picture way. She realized that her husband's affair wasn't her fault, and that the issues lay within him, not her. She stopped blaming herself and she started replacing negative self-talk with positive affirmations. With all of this came great freedom and release unlike anything Barbara had ever before experienced. In fact, she even released her husband before long. Just as she had let go of toxicity and tightness in her body, she also let go of it in her life and closest relationships.

After a while, this different way of seeing the world trickled into other areas of Barbara's life as well. She blamed herself less, felt more empowered, exercised her voice, gracefully released her emotions, and had a bigger-picture view of life, the world, and her place in it.

Get to Know Your Head

Every single person on this planet has to deal with gravity. This is particularly noteworthy when we talk about the head (which includes everything from your neck up to your cranium) because, on average, the human head weighs around thirty pounds. That's a lot of weight to hold up!

In my structural integration work, I often see people lose an entire inch of height simply due to the impact of gravity on their head and spine. As we've discussed, sitting leads to massive compression in the body. As a direct result of this, many—if not most—of us tend to subconsciously lean our head forward, which creates stagnation in the neck and throat.

This issue is exacerbated by the fact that most of us very rarely put much thought into the action of holding our head up. From a structural point of view, the weight of the head is partially being held up by the jaw and the base of the skull (technically known as the occipital bone). That's a lot of pressure weighing down on these two relatively delicate areas. Many of us tighten and clench our jaw and cranium when we begin to feel fatigue or fear—a locking motion that creates a lot of compression, tension, and blockage in the throat, jaw, neck, and cranium. Moreover, it inhibits cerebrospinal fluid (CSF) from flowing up and down our spine freely.

This clear liquid carries oxygen and sugar to the brain and removes carbon dioxide, waste, and toxins. This flow occurs because the bones of your sacrum and skull subtly move six to twelve times per minute, almost like they are floating in still water. Breathing also acts as a pump to propel CSF up the spine and around the brain. Anything that blocks this fluid flow messes with the proper circulation of CSF and can negatively affect the nervous system. Head and core tension block the flow of CSF.

But, wait! There's more. When our head drops forward—which happens often when we spend a lot of time looking down—the muscles in our neck are stretched out and weakened. Over time, this causes those muscles to become long-tight in the back and short-tight in the front—resulting in a saggy and weak neck. Our thyroid gland, which is located at the base of the front of our neck, can become clogged. Like all glands, the thyroid gland loves circulation, movement, and space, so it can become a potentially serious and widespread issue if it is congested, compressed, or blocked. The thyroid influences many of our most important organs, including our heart, brain, liver, kidneys, and skin. It impacts our metabolism and energy levels, among many other things.

Even our sinus canals take a hit from a tense, stressed, forward-leaning, and overthinking head. They become shorter, denser, and heavier, which affects our entire facial structure and causes the skin to sag. In my practice, when focusing on the head, neck, and jaw, I start by having my client lie on a 36-inch foam roller to see where the alignment is from the start. Then I look at where the head is in relation to the top of the neck, check the range of motion in the neck and jaw, and then share techniques for smoothing out the fascia, realigning the neck, and reactivating the strength in the neck muscles. I also help bring awareness to the tension in the jaw, noting how it's directly connected to the pelvic floor, and go over jaw relaxation techniques as well.

The Head and Holistic Health

Did you know that you can create more symmetry in your face simply by relaxing and creating more space in your jaw? Weird, but true.

The jaw mimics the hips on a structural level. For the same reasons that you want your hips to be fluid and light, it's important for your jaw to be free of tension. But just as many of us carry stress in our pelvic floor without even noticing it, the same is true of the jaw. We live in a constant state of clench and tightness, which can result in anything from generalized pain in the jaw area to intense headaches. Grinding our teeth and a clenched jaw go hand in hand. When we grind our teeth, a tight jaw begins to feel like status quo. Likewise, when your jaw is tight, the natural contraction of your muscles will cause your teeth to grind. A tight jaw can make your face appear caved in, droopy, sad, and wider and can even furrow your brow.

If you find yourself doing this, envision your neck as upright and elegant, elevating the crown of your head so that it reaches to the heavens, and holding your jaw parallel to the floor so that your chin is tilted neither up nor down. By simply seeing this in your mind's eye, you will find that you adjust and straighten, creating more space between your occipital bones, neck, and shoulders. A great way to create space, build strength, and realign the neck is by putting this posture into practice while you're driving. Lean your car seat an inch back, tuck your chin under, and gently press the base of your skull into the seat's headrest by using the back of the neck muscles. This will decompress your cervical spine, bring your jaw line back to a healthy position, and help release the jaw tension from the forward-head posture.

Many people have jammed up the fascia in their face, scalp, and neck to the extent that they have locked themselves into a state of constant, compressed tension. As a result, to move their head, they have to move their shoulders. The movement of head turning should originate from the cervical spine or neck. Ideally, you want a flexible, fluid, willowy "bobblehead" when you walk, like those hula girls that truck drivers have on their dashboards. Just like your hips and spine should undulate, so should your head. Your bones are not fused, they are sutured, which means they were not designed to be completely stagnant—they should have some flexibility.

The Throat, Third Eye, and Crown Chakra

The head is associated with not one, but three chakras: the throat chakra, third eye chakra, and crown chakra.

The throat chakra is associated with the color blue. It is all about communication, openness, honesty, and purity of speech. Through speech, we put into action our ability to make the right choices and exercise willpower and self-expression. We can think of speech as the crossover between our heart (the chakra directly below the throat) and the subconscious (located higher up in our head, in the third eye). Our voice allows us to express ourselves to the world, not only through our words, but also through our creativity.

The throat chakra includes the thyroid gland, which regulates body temperature and metabolism. In the Western world, we tend to think of metabolism through the lens of weight gain or loss. Metabolism does impact our weight, but, more importantly, it converts food into useful energy—in other words, life force.

The next chakra associated with this area is the third eye, located in the center of our forehead, between the eyes. When the third eye, represented by the color purple, is open and clear, we have insight, which allows us to see the difference between illusion and truth. It helps us to understand ourselves, others, life, and reality as they are. With this ability, we can make better decisions. Through the third eye, we obtain wisdom of all varieties, including mystical wisdom.

The third eye includes the pituitary gland, which is located near the base of the skull. The pituitary gland is a small organ, about the size of a pea. It sits at the base of the brain, produces many hormones, and is known as the master gland of the body.

These hormones are responsible for many bodily processes and for stimulating other glands to do their jobs well.

Also included here is the pineal gland, which releases the hormones that influence our body chemistry, such as melatonin, a hormone that affects our wake and sleep cycles. Many believe that the pineal gland is an alchemist, because it transmutes melatonin into some very profound, radical neurotransmitters that help heal and regulate the body.

Awakening the third eye gives us the power to see what might be, to see potential. It allows us to open up to our intuitive sensibility and inner perceptions, and to sense and visually interpret energy around us.

Finally, the crown chakra is associated with the color white. It governs information of both consciousness and the collective consciousness. This is considered a very mystical chakra, but we can also think about the crown in terms of getting out of our head and allowing ourselves to channel in creativity, inspiration, and information. When we let go of overthinking and the spiral that it creates, we open up space in our brain for all of the good stuff that the crown chakra has to offer.

It is here that we can connect to the universal source, open to giving and receiving energy, awareness, and information from both worldly and otherworldly sources. We can get in touch with our sacred and limitless nature.

The Head, Jaw, and the Pelvic Floor

The vagus nerve creates a direct line from our brain to the on/off stress button in the pelvic floor. Think of these as bookends of the body's power centers: the jaw and pelvic floor are both physiologically and emotionally connected. The alignment of one has a direct impact on the alignment of the other.

In my practice, I've seen that when my clients release fascial restrictions and reawaken the neuromuscular connections to their pelvic floor, their jaw will simultaneously move, stretch, and relax, mirroring the pelvic floor release. This connection is huge; it means when we can deepen our awareness and release one area of the body, we can also release in the other. Dentists and physical therapists have noticed this same connection, and have even done studies proving that it works both ways: when we improve mobility in the jaw, we unleash tension and promote power and strength in the pelvis, and vice versa.

Another commonly recognized connection is the cranial-sacral connection. Craniosacral work, which was developed by osteopath doctors, fuses together energy and body work. Although we think of the bones in our cranium as being fused, they're not (thus, the "soft spot" on babies' heads). On the contrary, there are sutures in the skull that not only have the capacity to move, but are actually meant to move. As we discussed earlier, this slight movement is essential for cerebral fluid to flow. When we clench our jaw enough over a period of time, we can actually tighten the fascia and the bones in our head. This results in a whole host of issues, ranging from tension headaches to an inability to create and connect.

When it comes to physical stress relief, I know a lot of people who swear by deep tissue massage. I love a good massage as much as the next person, but craniosacral work is actually far more effective when it comes to stress release, because it deals directly with the nervous system, which is the root of all tension or knots. Craniosacral work looks at the body as an energetic entity, decongesting stuck energy and bringing your nervous system into a more relaxed parasympathetic state. Rather than using the force that is applied through massage, craniosacral work is all about harnessing, allowing, and listening. It allows us to create space and get back into our natural, balanced energetic rhythm and rebalances the nervous system.

A craniosacral practitioner will help your energy flow in a gentle, pulsating, and healing manner. When done correctly, they will make clear the connectedness of your body in very real ways—for example, a practitioner might do work on your hip that you can quite literally feel on your jaw, just as clearly as if someone had their hands on your face. The overall impact of this is the ability to breathe more deeply. With deep breathing and softening, we are able to calm the nervous system and find a place of surrender. We can let go and become vulnerable. It is in this state that true, deep healing can occur.

In this place of rest-and-digest, we find the fountain of youth. We can heal and restore our tissues, our minds, our bodies, and our physical wounds and uncoil emotional wounds. It alleviates pain of all varieties, which is really just blockage.

The Head and Stress

When we release stress in our jaw, it has a holistic impact, thanks to the craniosacral connection. This release can ease us into a state of rest-and-digest, which is where we heal, rejuvenate, and energize on all levels—physical, mental, and emotional.

Even small measures of awareness and release impact the

nervous system in very meaningful ways. You don't have to be in a yoga or meditation class to transport yourself to a different, more low-key state—it can be accomplished on a moment-by-moment basis.

HEAD, NECK, AND JAW STRESS HYGIENE

To begin building new, nonreactive habits around stress, try this simple stress-combating exercise the next time you catch yourself in a moment of clutching.

Let your arms hang down as you are either standing or sitting. Reaching your right arm long, inhale as you tilt your head to the left. Exhale as you lift your chin up and then tuck the chin down to clear tension in the neck. Repeat on the other side and do 5 times each side.

Movement Medicine for the Head

Head and Neck Release with Bridge

Lie face-up on the mat and place the ball under the base of your skull. Inhale to fill up your lungs, and exhale as you soften down into the ball. Reach your arms long by your side with palms down. Inhale as you lift your hips and gently tuck your chin to decompress your neck. Exhale as you lower back down. Repeat this series of movements 8 times.

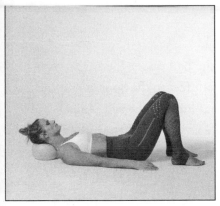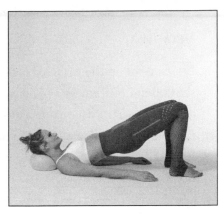

Head and Neck Release with Bridge

Neck Extension and Flexion

Lie face-up on the mat and place the ball under the base of your skull. Bend your knees and bring your feet to the floor, hips-width distance apart. Reach your hands down long by your side and inhale as you lift your chin up toward the ceiling. Exhale, tuck your chin, and lengthen the back of your neck, pressing your head down into the ball while you lift your ribs slightly to increase the traction in the back of your neck. Repeat this series of movements 8 times.

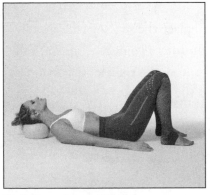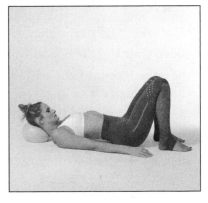

Neck Extension and Flexion

Neck Twist

Lie face-up on the mat and place the ball under the base of your skull. Bend your knees and bring your feet to the floor, hips-width distance apart. Reach your arms out long to the side. Inhale and turn your head to the right. Exhale as you turn your head to the left. Repeat this series of movements 8 times on each side.

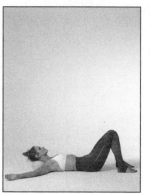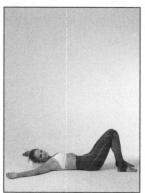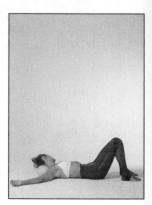

Neck Twist

Side-Lying Neck and Jaw Release

Come down on your right side and place the squishy ball directly above your right ear. Inhale as you rotate your gaze up and roll the sphere toward the back of your skull. Exhale as you twist your head and gaze down toward the floor as the ball massages the right side of your head. Return to your starting position and slowly open your mouth to stretch your jaw. Close your mouth. Repeat this series of movements 8 times on each side.

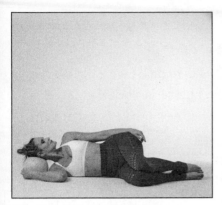
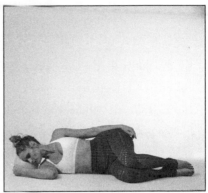

Side-Lying Neck and Jaw Release

Cranialsacral Release

Lie face-up on the mat and place the ball under the base of your skull. Bend your knees and bring your feet to the mat, hips-width distance apart. Reach your arms long by your sides, creating space in your spine. Come up into bridge position. Inhale as you tip your left hip down and right hip up, freeing up your sacrum. Exhale and lower your right hip down, left hip up. Alternate and repeat this series of movements 8 times on each side.

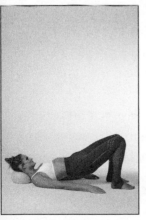
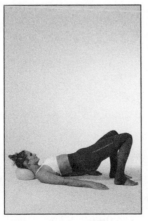
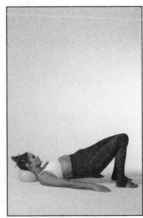

Cranialsacral Release

Pelvic Floor and Jaw Release

Sit on the ball, allowing your sitz bones to melt over it. Bring your first three fingers to the masseter jaw muscle, just below your cheekbone. Take an inhale and then on your next exhale bite down and clutch your pelvic floor. Next, inhale as you soften your pelvic floor over the ball and open and stretch your mouth. Slowly close your mouth, gently massaging your jaw muscles as you continue to open and close your mouth. Continue to massage for 30 to 60 seconds.

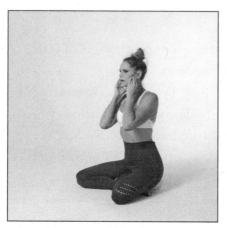 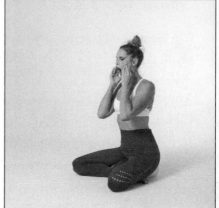

Pelvic Floor and Jaw Release

Ear Pulls

Sit on the ball, allowing your sitz bones to melt over it and your pelvic floor to soften. Take your first and second fingers and thumb and place them on the tops of your ears, as close to your head as possible. Inhale as you pull and stretch your ears by sliding your fingertips over the sides of your ears. Exhale and release. Repeat this series of movements 8 times.

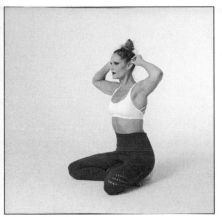

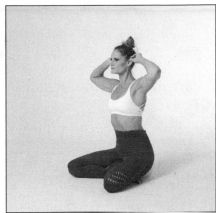

Ear Pulls

Temporalis Release

Take your first two fingers and place them behind your ears near your earlobe. Inhale as you slide the two fingers along your skull and up behind your ear. Exhale as you continue sliding up and simultaneously open and stretch your mouth and jaw. Once you

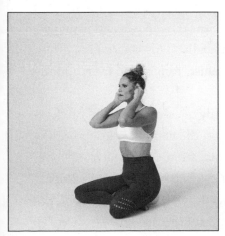

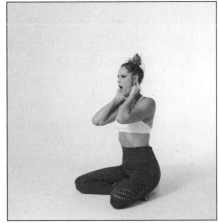

Temporalis Release

get to just above the ear, gently massage your temporalis muscle (located right above your ear) to release jaw and head tension.

Breathe into Your Head

Stand with your feet hips-width distance apart and soften your knees. Breathe naturally for a couple rounds of breath, noticing how it feels. On your next inhale, reach your arms out to the side and open them up to the sky. Open your chest and allow your rib cage to expand as you tilt your head back and look up to clear the thyroid gland and realign your neck. As you exhale, slowly lower your arms down by your side and let your chin drop toward your chest. Repeat this cycle of breath 10 times.

Heal and Balance Your Head

Ancient Ayurveda to Cleanse and Open

The neti pot is one of ancient Ayurveda's greatest gifts to the modern world. It helps clean and clear our sinuses and nasal passages, both physically and energetically. This is more important than ever, thanks to all of the exhaust, fumes, and overthinking we are exposed to on a daily basis.

The neti pot can be used on a daily or as-needed basis. By clearing blockage in the nose and sinuses, the neti pot helps us breathe more deeply; alleviates allergies; and, from a mystical standpoint, opens up the channels of the third eye to promote deeper clarity.

To use, fill a neti pot with warm water and ½ teaspoon sea salt. As you breathe through your mouth, place the spout at the opening of one nostril, and tilt your head to the side and slightly forward so that the water flows through that nostril and out the other side. Continue until the neti pot is empty, then refill and repeat on the other nostril. This can be a weird sensation at first, but remember to breathe through your mouth as you rinse, and over time you will get used to it and enjoy the benefits.

Pump Up Your Endorphins with a Song

Singing vibrates your throat and jaw area, releasing physical tension as well as endorphins, which are associated with pleasure. It also releases oxytocin, which enhances feelings of trust and bonding. This may explain why studies have found that singing decreases feelings of depression and loneliness. Recent research even points to the fact that music "evolved as a tool of social living." The pleasure we derive from singing is an evolutionary reward for coming together cooperatively rather than hiding out alone in our caves.

Singing (as well as humming and chanting) relieves tension, brings you into the present moment, and is a great way to channel emotion and clear energy. Science believes the benefits of singing are cumulative. To this point, singers have lower levels of cortisol, which indicates less stress. So make a habit of singing your heart out, baby!

Gua Sha

This ancient Chinese alternative therapy is designed to get stagnant chi moving, boost collagen, and flush stress and lines from the face. You can do a gua sha massage on yourself with the amazing rose quartz gua sha tool (I order mine from Odacite). Gently stroke it along your face to stimulate circulation and melt any density in your soft tissues. This will increase blood flow and even give your face a (naturally) lifted look. It smooths out wrinkles, removes dead skin, stimulates lymphatic drainage, boosts collagen, helps break up energy, and promotes healing.

Although this technique can be utilized on many areas of the body, I particularly enjoy using it on the face, jaw, and neck because of the uplifting and age-delaying benefits of boosting collagen and reducing tension. Gua sha is particularly effective for alleviating saggy jowls, under-eye bags, headaches, forehead frown lines, a tight jaw, and even neck pain.

TAKE A CLEARING CEREMONIAL BATH

This calming and soothing bath of sea salt and clary sage will help you unlock your intuitive knowledge and wisdom. This special blend will help calm your nervous system and relax your tissues so you have a super-restorative, restful night's sleep, which will dramatically release tension in your jaw, scalp, and face. It will inspire your imagination, usher your dreams into reality, and help you recognize yourself as the creator of your own life. You will emerge feeling soothed and open, connected to something higher than yourself, and with a more positive outlook on love and a clearer view of your own life path.

2 cups magnesium chloride salt
6 to 8 drops clary sage essential oil

Draw a warm bath and add the magnesium chloride salt and essential oil under the running water. Stir the water with your hand to incorporate the salt and oil throughout the bath.

Mantra and Visualization for the Head

"I am connected to myself and source. It is safe for me to assert and express my truth clearly, confidently, and with love."

Find a cross-legged seat in a comfortable position on your cushion, roller, or squishy ball. Allow your hips to relax, sitz bones to ground down, and your spine to float tall, so that it is effortlessly long. Imagine your life force traveling up and down your spine.

Shift your focus to your jaw area. Notice if you are clenching. Soften your tongue away from the roof of your mouth and allow your lower jaw to hang and be slack. Bring that awareness into your throat area and even under your ears. Soften the tension and holding.

Now turn your attention to your occipital bones at the base of your neck. See if you can soften here. Relax your inner ears, softening all of the muscles surrounding your ears, including your jaw attachment muscles. Move your awareness to the space behind your eyeballs, seeing if you can relax them. How about your forehead and eyebrows?

By softening in this area, we allow more space for intuition and inner knowing to be present and to flow. We can start to turn down the overthinking that results in so much pressure, both literally and figuratively.

Feel the energy coming up from your pelvis, along your spine, and allow it to soften your head. Deepen your awareness of sensation. How do you feel right now? What do you notice?

Keep relaxing the energy in your skull around your hairline, temples, and even right at the top of your head. Imagine a little halo of energy floating over your head, rising out of you and reaching up toward the sky.

Feel the expansion of your head energy. Feel it lighten, soften, and brighten. Notice if you have any thoughts or emotions that seem to be stuck. See if you can send those off or witness them like a movie, without getting caught up in the judgment of them.

The more you can open up to your true inner knowing, the less you will overthink and create stress. The more you will connect to your own creativity. The more you can allow inspiration to come in.

Feel the sensations of lightness, relaxation, and calm. Imprint this into your nervous system so that when you feel stress arise or overthinking kicks in, you can make an empowered choice not to bear down or hold on, but to soften the energy in your body. This allows you to soften your reaction.

Take a deep breath in and let it go. Feel the sensations of length and space and lightness, and an effortless sensation of lifting upward even as you are grounded and supported.

Activate Your Connecting Superpower Through the Head

When I work with clients who are dealing with pain from the top of their spine up through their head, I often find that they are too cerebral, too judgmental, unable to see things clearly, and overthinkers. They become so stuck in their head that other aspects of their being aren't flowing. They aren't feeling sensations in their bodies, their imaginations have been bogged down by the responsibilities of life, and they are not freely feeling, connecting to, or expressing their emotions.

When we swallow our emotions, they can manifest physically as a tight jaw, compressed sinuses, a frowning forehead, or headaches (including migraines). It blocks our chi from flowing. An overfixation on thinking, critiquing, judging, and subsequent emotional stagnation takes us out of the present moment. This is particularly prevalent in America. This has long been the case, but it's becoming worse as we are increasingly plugged into our devices, scrolling, analyzing, comparing, and processing more information.

Speaking our emotions in a safe place generally quiets the noise in our head. This idea is at the very crux of talk therapy, in which patients are often asked to discuss their worst fear or outcome. When we put voice to an emotion of any variety—and *especially* fear—we enjoy not only emotional freedom, but also physiological freedom.

Outside of a therapist's office, this usually translates to the ability to have open and honest conversations. As we all know, this is sometimes easier said than done. However, it's a skill we can all cultivate. Developing this ability also allows us to connect with others and, most of all, to connect with ourselves and what we are feeling at any given moment.

When we talk, we not only communicate and express our authentic feelings and emotions, but we also want to connect to the heart, which communicates with compassion. Language is a powerful tool, because words are one of our primary modes of connecting with others. Choosing our words consciously allows us to be more precise with our desires and to better connect both to others and to those things that are greater than ourselves.

Our daily communication with others and self-talk help shape our reality negatively or positively. Becoming conscious of the language we use to talk to ourselves helps us get to the root of what's blocking us from true transformation. When we become aware of how we are speaking about ourselves on a daily basis, we become more aware of how we can control our perceptions. It's a simple and powerful shift. Taking stock of the stories we tell ourselves is an incredible way of accessing the truth of our place in the world. We can speak honestly while still choosing our words intentionally. Integrating conscious language into our vocabulary is a great way to create shifts in our bodies and lives.

Conscious language puts into practice the idea that almost everything we say can be transformed into a message to the universe expressing our true desires. The words we choose can serve as an ongoing and consistent affirmation of what we want to bring into our lives and where we want to go. For example, you might say, "I choose to go to work," rather than "I have to go to work." Can you see how those two phrases land completely differently in your body? Or how does it feel to say, "I get to pick up my daughter from school," instead of "I have to go pick my daughter up"? Or what does it feel like to say, "I get to pay my bills" instead of "I have to pay my bills"? It really is a huge shift on every level.

These super-simple shifts take you into a vibrational state of feeling positive, present, and grateful in a split second. Try this when you send texts or emails as well. It's truly magical and super easy to start incorporating into your life. You will find yourself becoming more aware of, intentional, and impeccable with your words. When we choose our words carefully, we can live our lives in a more intentional way.

Not only does more flow and intention-based living come from speaking our truth—a sense of empowerment does as well. Speaking allows us to more easily create what we want, for the simple reason that it lets others know what we are thinking, feeling, and desiring. If you don't ask, you can't receive—or, at the very least, it makes it much more difficult to receive what you truly and deeply want.

Expression of words alone is not enough. We have to follow that up with action and accountability. Notice if your actions and reactions match your words. Are you actually living the life you're talking about? When these two sync up, magic happens.

ALTERNATIVE THERAPIES FOR THE HEAD

Aromatherapy

I absolutely love the Pure Calm Wellness Aromatherapy Oil by Uma Oils. It includes chamomile essential oil to calm tension and vetiver essential oil to help ground and center. This blend naturally helps you get out of your head and alleviates feelings of stress by promoting calmness from within. Put some in the diffuser or dab it on your temples to mentally unwind and reset your connection center. You can find this blend at www.umaoils.com.

Crystals

To heal your head, select the crystal that resonates with you most and place it on your third eye center (the space on your brow between the eyes). As it rests there, meditate, relax, or visualize the outcome you hope to receive. For a more consistent infusion of healing vibes, you can also carry your selected crystal with you in your purse or pocket, wear it as jewelry, or place it in your home or car.

- **Amethyst**—this third eye chakra stone taps you into personal wisdom and activates the power within
- **Clear quartz**—brings clarity in the mind and amplifies energy; expands consciousness and amplifies psychic abilities
- **Lapis lazuli**—the "stone of truth" restores the ability to communicate authentically and opens, stimulates, and balances the entire system
- **Turquoise**—stimulates and balances energy and removes negativity; restores the confidence to speak and express true feelings

Tea

Thyme and fennel are a powerful combination and also work well separately. Thyme is known as a spiritual herb. It opens up our ability to communicate and resonates with the throat chakra to allow us to speak with passion and purpose.

Thyme can be a miracle for banishing sore throats. This multifaceted herbal tea offers so many other benefits, too. Research has found that it can also be used to support healthy nervous, immune, respiratory, and digestive systems.

Fennel seeds are thought to be filled with natural compounds that can help decrease inflammation in the thyroid.

This tea can boost your immune system and help relax the autonomic nervous system and soft tissues. Plus, it's a lovely way to nurture your connecting power center. Sipping this brew assists us in achieving a state of being rather than doing. This spiritually enhancing infusion will help you connect with your higher self and find a place of calm, effortless knowing.

Add some fresh thyme and fennel seeds to your teapot, pour hot water over the herbal blend, and let it steep for 5 minutes. Add a teaspoon of Manuka honey to boost the soothing effects and, just like that, you have a super-healing tea to sip and enjoy!

Nourish Your Head

Herbs for the Head

A good supply of iodine is required to help your thyroid function optimally. Seaweed and kelp have been used by many ancient cultures to help increase iodine intake and balance thyroid function. Seaweed also contains many other essential nutrients and minerals that help the body. Your body and spirit will thank you for adding this sacred ocean vegetable to your diet.

Vitamins and Minerals for the Head

MAGNESIUM

While a nutrient-rich diet is the best way to prevent and alleviate headaches, an additional magnesium supplement can be quite helpful. People who frequently experience headaches tend to have low magnesium levels. Increasing those levels can naturally relieve headaches.

Doctors recommend taking between 200 and 600 milligrams of magnesium per day to prevent headaches. I like to take magnesium in powder form, because this is the most bioavailable way to ingest it. I take it at night before bed to have the deepest, most restorative sleep.

VITAMIN B12

Vitamin B12 is a crucial B vitamin that's essential for nerve tissue health, brain function, and the production of red blood cells. It plays a vital role in maintaining the myelin sheath, or covering, of the nerves. A diet deficient or insufficient in vitamin B12 may cause problems with the functioning of your nervous system. It's also a great tension-headache killer. Although B12 is found in fish, almonds, and sesame seeds, many of us still don't get our recommended daily dose of 2.4 micrograms.

A blood test can determine your B12 levels. A normal range is anywhere between 200 and 900 picograms per milliliter. Most experts agree that values less than 200 picograms per milliliter constitute a B12 deficiency.

Particularly if you suffer from frequent headaches, a B12 capsule a day may very well be an easy fix that has a significant impact on your life.

FOODS THAT AWAKEN AND HEAL THE HEAD

- **Blue foods**—blueberries, blue potatoes
- **Purple foods**—beets, blackberries, eggplant, plums, purple cabbage, purple carrots, purple grapes, purple kale
- **Brazil nuts** to balance thyroid
- **Chlorella** to help remove heavy metal toxins in the brain

Crown Tonic

MAKES 8 OUNCES

Turmeric is a powerful antioxidant and anti-inflammatory compound that is believed to have a ton of benefits for your brain, including improving memory and even helping new brain cells grow. This tonic is also bolstered by ginger, another anti-inflammatory and antioxidant that aids digestion and relieves nausea. Lemon will alkalize and help to boost your immune system, while cayenne (which assists in the bioavailability of turmeric) rounds this tonic out by boosting metabolism.

    1 tablespoon fresh grated turmeric or ½ teaspoon ground turmeric
    1 tablespoon fresh grated ginger or ½ teaspoon ground ginger
    Juice of 1 lemon, along with leftover peeled rind
    Cayenne
    3 cups filtered water

Add the turmeric, ginger, lemon juice and leftover lemon rind, cayenne, and filtered water to a small saucepan. Bring the mixture to a simmer over medium heat. Once the tonic begins to simmer, place a small strainer over serving glasses and divide the tonic between two or three servings. If the tonic is too potent for you, dilute with more hot or warm water.

Store leftover tonic in the refrigerator up to three days. To serve, reheat on the stovetop until it is just warm to avoid breaking down the major antioxidants.

Enlightening Elixir

MAKES 12 OUNCES

The pineal gland, which sits in the middle of our brain, is small but mighty. It's been linked to mental and physical well-being and even to spiritual connection. As of late, the modern lifestyle has created some congestion in this precious gland, which is contributed to by toxins from food and water, and even the stress hormones our bodies over-produce. The apple cider vinegar is in this elixir because it is thought to assist in detoxifying the pineal gland, while the leafy greens and parsley are full of cleansing chlorophyll, vitamins, minerals, and antioxidants. Lemons are a common and delicious ingredient that not only brighten the flavor, but also contain nutrients that can contribute to increasing oxygen levels, repairing damaged tissue, and boosting the immune system.

> 2 cups organic baby spinach leaves
> 1 cucumber, chopped
> 3 stems fresh parsley
> Juice of 1 lime or lemon
> 1 tablespoon apple cider vinegar
> 1 cup filtered water

Place the spinach, cucumber, parsley, lemon or lime juice, apple cider vinegar, and water into a blender. Blend until smooth.

Nourishing Turmeric Bone Broth

MAKES 3 QUARTS

Though it's low maintenance to prepare, this broth does take time to simmer. It's worth it, though! The healing benefits of nutrient-dense bone broths are quite incredible. From immunity support, detoxification, joint healing, and collagen production for skin to healing and restoration for the gut, simmering bones offers a huge array of benefits. Feel free to mix it up and add any additional veggies you are craving to the broth.

4 pounds organic beef bones
¼ cup apple cider vinegar
6 cloves garlic, crushed or whole
3 tablespoons fresh turmeric, grated
2 onions, chopped
2 cups celery, chopped
1 teaspoon cayenne pepper
4 sprigs fresh thyme
Himalayan salt, to taste

Place the beef bones, apple cider vinegar, garlic, turmeric, onions, celery, cayenne pepper, and thyme into a large pot over low heat. Simmer for 1 hour. Remove the excess foam and return the broth to a simmer for 9 to 10 more hours before tasting. Continue simmering until you reach your desired taste. Add a pinch or two of Himalayan salt if desired.

Once you're happy with the flavor of the broth, strain it through a sieve into glass containers or store the broth until you are ready to serve. Discard the strained bones and vegetables.

To serve, heat the broth and pour it into a small bowl. Add healing superfood herbs of your choice on top to taste. I particularly enjoy dandelion and calendula.

Bone broth can be stored in the fridge for up to 4 days and in the freezer for up to 1 year.

SHORTEN YOUR SIMMER TIME

Using an Instant Pot shortens the cooking process for bone broths from 9 hours to 2! This is a great investment to make for your well-being. Turning a pile of leftover bones and veggies into 3 quarts of beautiful, nourishing bone broth in just a few hours is truly priceless.

Conclusion

Congratulations on taking the first steps toward creating a more aligned, enjoyable, purposeful, and present life. Even if you haven't yet included a single practice contained in this book in your everyday life, by picking up this book you have made a choice to open your mind to change and more empowered choices. Like I said at the beginning: the biggest tasks before you are making a choice to change, becoming more aware of how you live your life, and recognizing the state you are in as it changes from moment to moment.

The most important thing you can do moving forward—more important than any single practice in this book—is taking the time to listen to yourself and your body. Notice what you need in any given moment. Notice how you feel. Listen to what your body needs. Notice where you can let go.

In the world today, we are taught to do, do, do, push, push, push, and achieve, achieve, achieve. For just a day, or even an hour, see if you can feel a little more, make choices from your heart, know we are all connected, and allow things to happen. With that, practice choosing your reaction as opposed to going into a subconscious pattern of stress and control. Harness the ability to ride the waves of life, rather than pushing upstream against it.

The difference between control and surrender is the difference between doing and being. Imagine for a moment how it would feel to get out of your own way, surrender into the feminine energy of being, and allow in all of the amazing things life has to offer.

Choose to be more present. All of the answers you need lie in the present and inside of you. So do freedom, fulfillment, connection, and joy. It is here that you will find true freedom—freedom in mind, body, heart, and space.

The best doctor is already within you. There is no replacement for cultivating a practice that heals, replenishes, and relaxes you from the inside out.

Acknowledgments

I am so grateful to the many individuals that have made this dream come to life. I am truly honored for the opportunity to share this healing knowledge I have spent my entire adult life pursuing with readers everywhere on the planet.

Thank you to my incredibly supportive husband, Gus Roxburgh, and our little mermaid girls for believing in me, constantly teaching me, and honoring my path, purpose, and passion.

Thank you to my mentors, my clients, our high-vibe-aligned tribe, my friends, and my family for the support, love, trust, and guidance you've given me along the way.

Thank you, Emmy Rossum, for sharing your journey to inspire a shift in perspective and motivate many to feel more empowered and aligned.

Thank you for the focused guidance of Leah Miller, my fabulous and gifted editor, and the wonderful team at Hachette and Grand Central Publishing.

Thanks also to Elise Loehnen; Kiki Koro; the visionary herself, Gwyneth Paltrow; and the whole team at *goop* for giving me such a powerful platform to share this empowering knowledge. I am forever grateful to my dear friend Michele Promaulayko for discovering me and uncovering my unique talent and writing my first article at *Women's Health* magazine back in the day.

A huge thank you to my incredible book agent Coleen O'Shea for helping me navigate the magical world of publishing and giving me the "tools" to share this knowledge. A huge thanks to the super-talented Nikki Van Noy for helping me put this knowledge into the right words so that I could communicate it in a simple, organized, and straightforward manner. Without these incredibly talented and generous people, this book would not have come to fruition.

Thank you to Annie McElwain, the talented photographer, for capturing these inspiring and helpful images.

Thank you to my dear and loyal clients for believing in me and trusting me. I'm so grateful to you all for allowing me to be creative and develop this program with your help—and of course for allowing me to test my theories on you! I am able to do what I do with passion and the knowledge that this program truly works only because of your constant support, enthusiasm, and encouragement.

Thanks to Dan, Steve, and Aimee for teaching me structural integration at the New School of Structural Integration. Thanks to Stacy Vargas and Sara Dacklin for inspiring me and teaching me true, pure classical Pilates.

Thanks to Sam Esmail, Baron Davis, Jarret Stoll, Molly Sims, Sarah Brokaw, Sophia Bush, Jenni Kayne, Melissa Rauch, and Gabby Reece for your guidance and support through the process of writing a book.

Thanks to my dad and Christie and my sister, Lindsey, and the rest of my family and friends for putting up with my ambition and drive.

I also want to acknowledge my late and much-loved mother, whose brave battle with cancer, which began when I was a teenager, provided the motivation to spend my life exploring this path of health and wellness.

Index

About the Author

One of the most sought-after alignment, fascia, and wellness experts on the planet, Lauren Roxburgh (Lo Rox), dubbed the Body Whisperer, is a bestselling author, the creator of her signature Lo Rox Aligned healing products, and the founder of the Aligned Life Studio subscription. Lo is trained in a wide variety of healing modalities, including Structural Integration, Pilates, Exercise Science, Athletic Training, and Yoga. Her method helps empower your entire being by helping you remove blockages in both the physical body and the emotional self. Her system helps align, sculpt, and slim thick, dense, and congested areas, actually reshaping your body. Ultimately her method will help you learn a new way of caring for yourself by releasing stress and fears, breathing more deeply, banishing tension and pain, strengthening your core and intrinsic muscles, rejuvenating your pelvic floor, and helping you expand and grow into your best self.